The Medically
Complex Child

THE MEDICALLY COMPLEX CHILD

The Transition to Home Care

Edited by

Neil J. Hochstadt, Ph.D.
La Rabida Children's Hospital and Research Center;
Department of Pediatrics, Pritzker School of Medicine
University of Chicago

and

Diane M. Yost, MSW
Illinois Department of Children and Family Services
Chicago

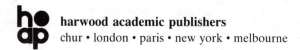
harwood academic publishers
chur • london • paris • new york • melbourne

92-61

Harwood Academic Publishers

Post Office Box 197
London WC2E 9PX
United Kingdom

58, rue Lhomond
75005 Paris
France

Post Office Box 786
Cooper Station
New York, New York 10276
United States of America

Private Bag 8
Camberwell, Victoria 3124
Australia

Library of Congress Cataloging-in-Publication Data

The Medically complex child : the transition to home care / edited by
    Neil J. Hochstadt and Diane M. Yost.
        p.   cm.
    ISBN 3-7186-0520-1 (case). — ISBN 3-7186-0521-X (paper)
    1. Chronically ill children—Home care.   2. Foster home care.
    3. Chronically ill children—Services for.   I. Hochstadt, Neil J.,
    1946–   .   II. Yost, Diane M., 1947–   .
    [DNLM: 1. Chronic Diseases—in infancy & childhood.   2. Home Care
    Services.   3. Home Nursing.   4. Social work.   WS 200 M4895]
    RJ380.M43   1991
    362.1'9892—dc20
    DNLM/DLC
    for Library of Congress   90-4876
                                                                            CIP

CONTENTS

SECTION VII OTHER CRITICAL ISSUES: LEGAL, ETHICAL AND FUNDING

SECTION VIII OUTCOMES

SECTION IX RESOURCES

FOREWORD

Throughout most of history, individuals who were ill have been cared for in the context of their family unit. Only in recent times have we seen the transfer of that responsibility to health care institutions. This change has come about largely as a result of the proliferation of hospitals and the explosion of new scientific technologies which have brought about so many lifesaving remedies for a wide variety of conditions.

In the face of these dramatic events, it became increasingly apparent that a growing number of individuals would survive with long-term conditions, and this led to the emergence of a new set of issues. Principal among them is how to orchestrate the care of the survivors who continue to have medically complex needs. Concern about this issue is especially critical for children because of the clear-cut evidence that a normalized environment is a prerequisite to their successful growth and development. While adults who acquire the need for intensive medical services have a lifetime of normal experiences to call upon during their rehabilitation, children who have continuing need for intensive medical care do not. It is clear that their long-term maturation and adjustment are severely threatened by spending large segments of their childhood away from a family and community setting.

Home care is a major alternative to the long-term hospitalization of children with medically complex conditions. The goal of home care is to maintain a balance between the child's medical, psychological and social needs by normalizing the child's life in a noninstitutional setting. This cannot be accomplished without a rather fundamental change in both the site and focus of care. It is predicated on a partial transfer of responsibility from the health care system to the family and community. This requires a change in the organization of the service package from one that is dictated entirely by medical needs to one in which family values and full participation in community life are emphasized as much for medically complex children as they are for healthy children. Although the objective is to make this transfer within the dictates of safe medical practice, home care inevitably includes taking a small degree of risk in order to obtain a large degree of benefit.

Pediatric home care programs have been successfully implemented in many sites around the country, and we now know that such care can be medically safe and that it affords significant emotional and developmental benefits. It is also clear that, under some circumstances, home care may result in a reduction of medical costs; but this alone should never be the basis for deciding for or against home care. Implementation of effective home care requires a major commitment of time and resources and the support of many individuals and systems that are not universally available and often inadequately reimbursed. Thus, home care may not be optimal or even possible for every medically complex child and every family.

Much of the recent growth of the health care establishment has been driven by a deep belief in the benefits, and even the supremacy, of medical science. Families whose children have been the beneficiaries of its "miracles," and providers who have devoted their professional lives to care within the system, may have a hard time refocusing their energies on the transition away from the medical institution. Shifting the paradigm to provide the balance necessary for successful home care requires the willingness to make major changes in traditional services and well-entrenched attitudes. This is not an easy transition either for families or providers. However, it must be navigated in order to form the cohesive partnership between professionals and families that is the key to successful long-term care in the home.

Neil Hochstadt and Diane Yost have put together this volume in the hope that it will serve to pave the way for many more children with medically complex conditions to make a successful transition to home care. They have undertaken the development of a practical guide to many of the issues that must be faced in the process of implementing an effective home care plan for a child and family. As such, this book represents an important milestone in helping to curtail unnecessary long-term institutionalization and in maximizing the opportunity for youngsters with serious ongoing health care needs to become productive and fulfilled members of our society.

Ruth E.K. Stein, M.D.
Professor of Pediatrics
Albert Einstein College of Medicine
Bronx, New York

PREFACE

The transition of medically complex children from hospital care to home care is one of the most challenging issues facing families and providers of health care and social services today. Having worked in this field for a number of years we were both struck by the fact that there were few, if any, books available to assist parents, caretakers, health care providers and child welfare personnel who work with medically complex children. Virtually all pediatric hospitals and child welfare agencies in the United States are struggling with the problem of developing appropriate techniques, mechanisms and resources to assist with the transition of medically complex children into the community; yet, despite this need, a central source of information does not exist. It is our intent to provide the many professionals and caretakers working in this area with a comprehensive overview of the most current issues, programs, approaches and resources available.

To achieve this goal many of the foremost authorities in this newly emerging field have contributed to this book. The diversity amongst contributors mirrors the interdisciplinary effort needed to transition these children to community care. This book is designed for *all* those working with the range of medically complex children. Biological parents will find it extremely valuable. Additionally, it places special emphasis on those medically complex children going to alternative care settings such as foster care or adoptive homes.

A variety of terms such as "medically complex", "medically fragile", and "technology-dependent" have been used to describe this diverse population of children. At the present time, there is no universally accepted terminology, nor are there accepted criteria. Some stress the reliance upon life-sustaining medical technology and devices; others stress the reliance upon highly skilled nursing care. These terminological problems are highlighted by the use of the terms "medically fragile" or "technology-dependent" when referring to a relatively stable subset of this population requiring only highly skilled nursing care or highly trained caretakers. Similarly, some of these children are only partially dependent upon technology, e.g., those children requiring mechanical ventilation for only part of the day. In point of fact, the different terminology used to attempt to define these children merely mirrors the diverse nature of disorders and treatment requirements of this population.

We faced several challenges in developing this book, including the heterogeneity of medically complex children, the diversity of treatment regimens and the fact that many different professions are involved in their care. Further complicating this situation is the fact that the number of medically complex children is rapidly growing. This is a reflection of the technological advances in medical care whereby many more children are being rescued through "high-tech" interventions. Additionally, other children with complex health care problems are surviving for longer periods of time. This population includes extremely low birth weight infants with complex medical sequelae, children who have suffered injuries secondary to child abuse and neglect and children with congenital and/or chronic disorders (including those children who are HIV positive). It is estimated by the Office of Technology Assessment of the United States Congress that ten percent of all chronically ill children are medically or technology dependent (chronically ill children comprise approximately ten percent of all children). Currently, there are more than 17,000 children who require ventilator assistance, parenteral nutrition, prolonged use of intravenous drugs or other device-based respiratory or nutritional support. There are an additional 80,000 children requiring constant monitoring, renal dialysis and device-assisted nursing care. This population continues to grow as does the need to develop techniques to transition and maintain these children in their homes or in community-based alternative care.

The benefits of home care for many of these children have become increasingly apparent. As the technology for their care becomes more manageable and accessible to parents and caretakers, attention can be turned to enhancing the cognitive and emotional development of these children. Even the best hospital environment cannot provide the warmth, support, and nurturing found in a home.

Additionally, changes in the economics of medical care and governmental regulations have caused us to re-evaluate our concepts of where children can and should receive medical care. Children who previously remained hospitalized for extended periods of time are now considered candidates for home care. While many of these children return to their biological families, a growing number require foster care or adoption services from an already over-taxed child welfare system because their biological parents or extended family are unwilling or unable to provide the requisite home care. Some examples of why medically complex children may enter foster/alternative care include: parental homelessness, parental mental illness or drug dependence and parents who are physically or cognitively incapable of caring for a child with complex home health care needs.

For the convenience of the reader, this book is divided into a number of sections. The introductory section provides an overview of the implications of medical technology and of the developing practice of specialized family foster care. The section on medical care provides an overview of the most prevalent medical conditions found in this population of children. It also provides an outline of the home health care tasks facing caretakers for each medical condition. In the same section, the role of the pediatric transitional unit in the management and transition of children to home care is reviewed.

The next section looks at the critical issue of discharge planning and the role played by nursing in this process. The section of psychosocial issues explores the contributions of social service providers and child welfare personnel to the transition process. In the same section, essential and pragmatic information regarding access to educational services is provided. The section on parenting medically complex children provides a unique perspective in that both chapters are authored by parents (foster and adoptive) of medically complex children. Both the Prybyls and the Geisslers give a first-hand account of the entire spectrum of transitional care, i.e., from the decision to care for a medically complex child through training and discharge planning to long-term home care.

The next section provides the readers with an overview of five innovative models of specialized care developed throughout the country. The uniqueness of each of these programs attests to the heterogeneity of this population of children and to the fact that these children and their caretakers require innovative and creative approaches. It is important to keep in mind that no single program can meet all of the needs of each child and family. Moreover, their needs are ever changing and evolving. As a result, care for these children requires a continuum of services—with access to the entire spectrum being required. As the conditions and needs of the child change, the need for services will most certainly change as well. Similarly, the family's requirement for services along the continuum will change as they become more proficient. This interface between the child's requirements, the family's needs, and the availability of services must be viewed on a matrix rather than on a linear dimension. It is one of the achievements (some would say miracles) of our age that we can think in these terms and devise these deliberate and hopeful strategies for the care of medically-complex children.

Legal, ethical and funding issues are addressed in the next section. A chapter is devoted to the increasingly important questions of entitlements and legal advocacy. As the rapidity of changes in medical technology outstrip our ability to integrate them, ethical issues become the nexus for the dialogue about our use of these technologies. Similarly, issues of public policy and the financing of care for this growing population of children are discussed in a separate chapter.

One of the few studies to have looked at how families who have cared for medically complex children have fared is reported on in the section entitled "Outcomes". The last section is a resource directory of the many agencies, programs, services and demonstration projects providing services to medically complex children and their families. The many resources in this directory attest to the wide range of agencies and professionals involved in the care of medically complex children. To the best of our knowledge, this directory is the only compendium of resources available for medically complex children.

Until recently, the pace of advances in medical technology has surpassed the ability of families, the child welfare system, the community and public policy to respond to needs of these children. This book demonstrates that innovative responses are beginning to identify barriers, redesign service delivery systems and ultimately close the gap between medical technology and our ability to care for medically complex children in the community.

Neil J. Hochstadt
Diane M. Yost

ACKNOWLEDGEMENTS

We would like to extend our thanks to the contributors to this volume for their willingness to share their expertise and for their receptiveness to editorial feedback. A special acknowledgement goes to Lorraine Halderman, administrative assistant; Shirley Cooks, secretary; and Joyce Anderson, secretary, whose clerical assistance was invaluable. The central figures of this book remain the caretakers—biological, foster and adoptive—without whose extraordinary commitment home care for this special population of children would not be possible.

CONTRIBUTORS

Gary R. Anderson, Associate Professor, Hunter College School of Social Work, City University of New York.

Legertha Barner, Child Welfare Specialist, Illinois Department of Children and Family Services, Chicago.

Terry Heintz Caldwell, Education Consultant, National Maternal and Child Health Resource Center, Children's Hospital, New Orleans, LA; New Orleans Public Schools, LA.

Phyllis Charles, Children's Home and Aid Society of Illinois, Chicago.

Leslie L. Clarke, Research Assistant, Center for Health Policy Research, University of Florida, Jacksonville.

Patricia H. Foster, Chairman, Department of Nursing, College of Health, University of North Florida, Jacksonville.

Deborah E. Fraze, Prescribed Pediatric Extended Care, Inc., Tampa, FL.

Steve A. Freedman, Director, Institute for Child Health Policy and National Center for Policy Coordination in Maternal and Child Health; Associate Professor of Pediatrics and Health Administration, University of Florida, Jacksonville.

Judith Geissler and Evan Geissler, Chicago, IL.

Phyllis Gurdin, Director, Specialized Foster Care, Leake and Watts Children's Home, Yonkers, NY.

Neil J. Hochstadt, Director, Behavioral Sciences Department, La Rabida Children's Hospital and Research Center; Associate Professor of Clinical Pediatrics, Department of Pediatrics, Pritzker School of Medicine, University of Chicago, IL.

Ann Holman, Coordinator, Psychosocial Team, La Rabida Children's Hospital and Research Center, Chicago, IL.

Paula Keinberger Jaudes, Associate Professor of Clinical Pediatrics; Chief, Section of Chronic Disease, University of Chicago, Pritzker School of Medicine; Associate Director, La Rabida Children's Hospital and Research Center, Chicago, IL.

Kathryn Kirkhart, Clinical Psychologist, Private Practice, New Orleans, LA.

Arthur F. Kohrman, Professor, Department of Pediatrics, University of Chicago; Director, La Rabida Children's Hospital and Research Center, Chicago, IL.

John Lantos, Assistant Professor, Departments of Pediatrics and Medicine, University of Chicago; Chief of the Medical Staff, La Rabida Children's Hospital and Research Center; Assistant Director, The Clinical Medical Ethics Center, University of Chicago, IL.

Donna G. Lester, Prescribed Pediatric Extended Care, Inc., Tampa, FL.

Mark J. Merkens, Adjunct Associate Professor, Department of Pediatrics, Oregon Health Sciences University, Portland, OR.

Sara Miranda, Director, Downs Syndrome Clinic, The Children's Hospital, Boston, MA.

Kathleen E. Murphy, Private Practice in Psychotherapy and Consultation, Glenview, IL.

Patricia M. Pierce, President, Prescribed Pediatric Extended Care, Inc., Tampa, FL.

Lynn Prybyl and Tom Prybyl, Chicago, IL.

Jane Quinton, Executive Director, Project Impact, Boston, MA.

Ruth E.K. Stein, Professor of Pediatrics and Director, Division of Pediatric Ambulatory Care, Albert Einstein College of Medicine of Yeshiva University, Bronx, NY.

Susan Sullivan-Bolyai, Continuity of Care Coordinator, La Rabida Children's Hospital and Research Center, Chicago, IL.

Jake Terpstra, Specialist, Family Foster Care, Child Care Institutions and Licensing, Children's Bureau, US Department of Health and Human Services, Washington, DC.

Mark Weber, Associate Professor of Law, De Paul University, College of Law, Chicago, IL.

J.M. Whitworth, Executive Medical Director, Children's Crisis Center, Inc., Jacksonville, FL; Associate Professor of Pediatrics, University of Florida, Jacksonville.

Diane M. Yost, Associate Deputy Director, Division of Policy and Plans, Illinois Department of Children and Family Services, Chicago.

Section I
Introduction

CHAPTER 1

MEDICAL TECHNOLOGY: IMPLICATIONS FOR HEALTH AND SOCIAL SERVICE PROVIDERS

ARTHUR F. KOHRMAN

The proliferation of medical technologies in the last two decades has presented medicine and social services with a new set of challenges: even as more and more is possible, and children survive who had no hope of doing so twenty years ago, new problems in their care, new ethical choices, new demands on professionals and social and medical systems have also proliferated. We can now keep alive the smallest and most dependent of infants, and the most severely impaired victims of congenital disorders, disease or trauma. Now, we must find ways of caring for those who continue to be dependent, constantly or intermittently, on the very technologies which have permitted their continued existence. It has become evident that they cannot and should not remain in the acute-care hospitals where resources for complicated care have traditionally been concentrated. Until relatively recently, the idea of moving technology-dependent children out of those hospitals into home or home-like settings was unthinkable; yet, it is equally unacceptable that they should spend their entire lives in hospitals or other institutions. Driven both by humane interests for returning children to the nurturing environment of families and by concerns for the immense costs of continued hospitalization, we have begun to devise systems for such movement; in the process we have become aware—sometimes painfully—of the consequences of the new adventure of home care for technology-dependent and medically complex children.

It is not only the increased sophistication of medical technologies and their applications that have led to the increasing numbers of children for whom complex home-care plans must be made. The rate of premature delivery, with its consequence of low-birth-weight infants with all their problems, continues high, and even is rising among the poor and in the inner cities. There are increased numbers of child victims of trauma, and with those numbers, more children who survive trauma with permanent or long-term incapacity and dependence on various technologies. Improved medical and surgical therapies have allowed more children with congenital anomalies and genetic diseases to survive longer; for many of them, however, survival carries with it a prolonged period of reliance on technology, and increased demands on families and other social supports, public and private. Because these children are living longer, their aggregate number in the population is steadily growing and the aggregate burden on support systems, both familial and societal, grows too.

While the care of many of these children might daunt even the most stable and financially secure of families, the special problems of those populations of medically-complex children who come from inner-city, often poor families are particularly vexing. The high correlation of poverty, single-parent families and very young maternal age with premature delivery and low birth weight results in a growing population of young children with multiple care needs for whom the family resources are least adequate; paradoxically, the very children who need the most have the least available. Similarly, trauma, both accidental and intentional, occurs much more frequently among the poor and those with already marginal families. Thus, many factors conspire to place the greatest burdens on those families and groups least capable of responding to the multiple critical needs, both medical and developmental, of medically complex children.

At the same time that the numbers of medically-complex children are increasing, the institutions in which children have traditionally been cared for are also undergoing drastic changes. Propelled by concerns about cost containment, with new capabilities to treat children formerly requiring hospitalization in outpatient settings, and with increasing use of hospital beds for extremely ill children and those who can benefit from new technologies such as organ transplant, acute-care children's hospitals have changed their missions, capabilities and staff patterns. Supportive services, such as social service and child life, have given way, and are often the most vulnerable to reduction in the face of budget constraints. Rehabilitative therapies are more and more found in specialty centers or in outpatient settings. The atmosphere of the contemporary children's hospital is much more geared to critically ill children, who require intensive acute care. Crisis abounds, and the problems of convalescence in the classical sense, and concerns about the social, cognitive and emotional development of child patients are relegated to outpatient settings or not attended to at all. Alternative inpatient settings for the care of medically-complex children are in short supply; only a very few children's hospitals in the United States are true transitional settings, and traditional children's long-term care institutions (the few that exist) are structured to care either for those unfortunate children with little or no developmental potential or for those who require minimal ongoing medical services.

Children who are medically complex, who have multiple service needs, and for whom detailed and lengthy discharge planning is the only route to successful home placement increasingly have no appropriate institutional base for the coordination of their care. The contemporary acute-care children's hospital is a frenzied, frightening place. The stabilized medically complex child and his or her family are confronted with the crisis of cardiac arrests, desperately sick children, stressed nursing and medical staffs; the urgent (and very real) priorities of the very sick children who increasingly occupy acute-care children's hospitals displace the less urgent but extremely important needs of the child with long-term illness or disability.

With the reordering of the priorities of acute-care children's hospitals, and with the growth of the population of children with long-term and complex needs for care, it becomes imperative that the child health care community seek and shape alternative institutions and programs to better meet the needs of those children, their families and caretakers. There are three major elements of a comprehensive system of care for medically-complex children to be addressed: (1), institutions where appropriate discharge planning and preparation can take place; (2), case-management programs to coordinate services and care for the child once discharged to home; and (3), continuing and effective support systems for the caretaking families, who most often *are* the case managers. A fourth critical element for the care of the growing numbers of medically-complex children who cannot, temporarily or permanently, go home to their biological families is a rational foster-care system, with close coordination between medical and social service systems; much of this volume is directed to that concern.

HOSPITALS AND PROFESSIONALS

Most medically complex children will have required care in an intensive-care unit, or have undergone extensive acute-care interventions at the outset of their lives or their illness. For these children, obviously, the acute-care hospital is a necessary and appropriate setting until the primary condition is stabilized; that is, until there is no longer a need for moment-to-moment or day-to-day adjustment in therapies and no dramatic interventions are anticipated. Other children will need a complex care plan as a result of loss of function or deterioration with the progression of a long-standing but slow-moving chronic illness, or because of an exacerbation of a chronic illness which is not seriously disabling during most of its course. For all of these children, a transitional hospital setting in which programs and staff are focussed on the long-term needs of the child and family is preferable to the traditional acute-care hospital, with its necessary attention to the crises of the seriously acutely ill child. The transitional hospital also should be available to serve when medically complex children discharged to home need rehospitalization, either as a planned reassessment or in cases of intercurrent illness or temporary changes in the family's capabilities to safely sustain the care program. The transitional hospital may also need to be available for respite for beleaguered families; while this is not a desirable use of a hospital setting, the absence of respite services in the United States at the present time often leaves no alternative.

The importance of respite for families who care for medically-complex children cannot be exaggerated; all families have times when there are greater demands than resources. A generally satisfactory home-care situation for a medically-complex child may become temporarily inadequate at such times of stress; a short period of respite, with the child either remaining in the home or moving to an alternate site, may allow the family to regain its competence and resume effective care of the child. Ideally, there should exist facilities, such as small group homes, where medically-complex children can reside under expert care while awaiting completion of discharge plan details, or the recruitment and training of foster families, or to provide short periods of respite for their primary caretakers. Unless and until such facilities are developed in this country, it will be necessary for hospitals to assume many of those responsibilities; clearly, the transitional hospital setting, as described in a subsequent section of this volume, is preferable to a typical acute-care hospital. Other sections of this book will describe very innovative programs designed to meet many of these needs. Unfortunately, these creative and successful programs are not widely available.

The possibility that children with complex medical needs may be cared for in settings other than the acute-care hospital, with all its technological capabilities, specialized personnel and emergency back-up systems, confronts medical professionals and medical administrators with the need to revise many of their traditional senses of responsibility, accountability and risk management. As discussed in a later chapter, home care for medically-complex children requires the sharing of risks with families and caretakers, in settings where the usual fall-back rescue systems are not present. Obviously, one of the goals of comprehensive successful discharge planning is to reduce risk to the child at home to the very minimum; nonetheless, the sharing of risks with families is unfamiliar to most hospital-based and trained physicians and nurses, and they may attempt to unnecessarily prolong the preparation period for discharge unless they have explicitly grappled with the new paradigm and accepted its implications.

ISSUES IN CASE MANAGEMENT

While there is general agreement that coordinated case management is essential to the success of home care programs for medically complex children, there are many different conceptualizations of case management and of the ideal case manager. (For the purposes of this discussion, case management does *not* mean simply the management of expenditure and control of dispensation of services, a construction used by many insurance companies and other payors.) There are many possible successful configurations for case management programs, either directed from within the discharging or transitional hospital or from without. However, an underexamined but critical issue, especially for social service providers, is the frequent assumption by most program planners that the parent will be the ultimate case manager. While it appears on the surface to be most logical to prepare the parent or foster parent to perform as the child's case manager, there are many pitfalls in that assumption which deserve scrutiny before the parent is vested with all responsibility.

There are many benefits in caring for a chronically ill or dependent child at home. The general reduction of anxiety of both child and caretakers with a shift in focus from illness and helplessness to recovery and function is dramatic. Significant physical and psychological improvements are seen in nearly all medically complex children whose care is transferred to the home setting. The familiar routines of family interaction have curative and enhancing powers in themselves. The reduction in the numbers of strangers and caretakers helps to reestablish attachments which were severely strained, or, for the infant, never made in the first place.

Many positive effects also potentially exist for the caretakers. However, the inevitable anxieties attendant upon receiving a child with complex needs at home may compromise or even totally negate the advantages. The caretakers must be helped to overcome the natural and inevitable worries of their new and potentially frightening situation, or the best planned home care program may appear overwhelming; with the result of readmission to the hospital for the child, accompanied by guilt and a deep sense of failure for the parents. Observations of many families over the last several years has permitted identification of some of the critical factors in the success of a home care plan, and some of the problems created in bringing a medically-complex child home. Anticipation of these may help professional providers to better prepare the caretaker family and to recognize and address potentially damaging problems in time to avert disintegration of the home care plan.

BARRIERS TO SUCCESSFUL HOME CARE

Role Confusion

Family members ordinarily provide care for other members, in ways that are usually carefully limited and reciprocal; they usually do not include (except for infants and small children) care of intimate functions. When acute illness or temporary disability requires temporary breaking of the informal rules of mutual care in a family, it is understood that the rules will be reestablished when the acute episode is over. It is with that understanding that illness-imposed dependency is tolerable for the sick person. Forced dependency on others, particularly family members, is appropriately resisted by most growing children, as a manifestation of their individuation and increasing independence. At the same time, companionship, familiarity, intimacy, solace—the critical and indispensable elements of family relationships—must be maintained. Indeed, these are the elements in home care which are most essential to the stability and progress of the compromised child. However, home care of the medically complex child creates the possibility of serious role conflict, in that the caretakers are often required to continuously breach the boundaries of intimacy and independence, often need to inflict pain in the course of providing care, and, at the same time are asked to confront the child's anger and despair. The caretakers of a medically complex child at home usually control the very technologies and perform the very procedures which are the sources of pain and anxiety for the child. The child thus sees essential and indispensable sources of comfort become the very carriers of anxiety and inflicters of pain. For the caretakers, this situation creates important conflicts; they must provide solace for the very anxiety and pain they have caused. The child may confuse the comforter with the tormentor; yet the child must also turn for reassurance to those who are causing psychological and, in many cases, physical discomfort.

There is also the possibility that the relationship between the child and the caretakers may become a provider-client or master-slave relationship; the normal developmental encouragement and support expected of the parent or foster parent may be obliterated as the caretaker focuses on the instrumental rather than on the affective tasks. A particularly difficult situation exists when the child is the first-born; the parents have no confidence or experience with their own basic child-rearing skills, even as they are confronted with a child with extraordinary demands for care and support.

Loss of Privacy

The caretakers of the medically complex child at home understandably have great anxiety about the functioning of technical support systems. They are inexperienced in differentiating normal from abnormal, and uncertain about when to become alarmed. As a consequence, the child may never be left alone or unstimulated by inquiring voices, caring touches or questions. Loss of privacy for caretakers is also a serious problem. The child's frequent probing "Are you there?" not only traps the parents but also feeds anxiety or guilt about not being available for events of consequence. Parents and caretakers often feel that they must hide the strains and passions of everyday life from the child and others—professionals and volunteers—in the environment. They are embarrassed and reluctant to openly demonstrate affection or disagreement; thus the parents' or caretakers' own affective relationships may be seriously compromised. The need for in-home support services compounds this problem.

Exhaustion

The many new and sometimes frightening tasks required of parents or caretakers are draining. They require constant attention, energy and organization. The organization and logistics of management of the medically complex child at home is time and energy demanding and may be confusing to those without managerial skills or previous experience. Uncertainties about fiscal management and the timely flow of payments add to the burden. Even when payments are adequate and prompt, there is a myriad of tiresome nagging and endless details, such as filling out forms, making phone calls to insure follow-through, waiting for and writing checks.

The physical demands of the child's care may also be significant. Transferring and positioning the child, moving equipment, giving treatments (such as physical and respiratory therapies), feeding and personal care all demand physical effort and often much strength. Parents and caretakers need to be helped to find ways to conserve their energies and to organize the tasks before them. They must also be reassured that fatigue is common and not a sign of impending failure. Most important, they should be given permission and encouragement to seek respite for themselves; specific respite plans for caretakers should be part of the final discharge plan.

Guilt

Parents repeatedly search their past actions and behaviors for some role they might have played in the causation of their child's plight—"What could or should I/we have done to keep this from having happened?" Clearly, foster parents of the medically complex child should not have guilt about causality, but even for them, as for biological parents, the intricacies of each of the many therapies and the vulnerability of the child together guarantee that some errors, some slips in technique will occur. Daily events in the care of a medically-complex child thus can create many opportunities for the caretakers to become guilty about their performance, or to reinforce longer standing guilts. That the caretakers or parents should feel such guilt is not unexpected; anticipation and discussion with the caretakers as part of the discharge process may prevent guilt from mounting to the level that it interferes with or compromises the child's care.

Endlessness

The medically complex child with chronic illness or disability usually improves slowly and has an unrelenting need for continuous therapies and services. Those realities, with the prospect of many years or decades—even a lifetime—of dedication of the family's resources and energy, can lead to a sense of despair and hopelessness. After they are learned and rehearsed, the routines of daily care become neither fearful nor novel. When the child has limited activity or interactive capabilities, the possibilities for new, creative interactions are limited. Caretakers may feel that they are trapped in a web of unrelenting demands, with little reward now or likely in the future. At the same time, siblings may find their world constrained by their parents' singular attention to a medically complex child. Children who are old enough to understand the demands which their illness or disability has imposed upon the family, may also become depressed as they realize that their problems have caused their loved ones unhappiness and limitation of opportunity. All members of the family may join in the perception that "there is no way out."

Continuing financial worries are among the most nagging and erosive problems. Because so many medically complex children are discharged to home with complicated and often inadequate and/or uncertain funding arrangements, concerns about money are likely to be a constant presence. The presence of a chronically disabled person in the home may severely restrict job mobility for the primary wage-earner in addition to necessitating that one family member forego earning opportunities. Thus, opportunities for improvement of earning capability may have to be sacrificed. Such monetary issues can only add to the sense of oppression and endlessness in the family which is disposed towards such feelings. These problems must be addressed head-on by the professionals arranging for and following the home care program.

CONCERNS ABOUT THE FUTURE

Home care for medically complex children is a relatively new venture; there are few data available about outcomes, either for the children or their caretakers. Relatively few medically complex children have resided in the care of foster families for extended periods. Much remains to be learned. While we know some of the anxieties and uncertainties for these patients and their families, and can guess at others, it is likely that many problems, not now clearly seen or anticipated, will become evident as more children with a wider variety of conditions are moved from hospitals to home. New issues will emerge, such as care for medically-complex children as their parents age, and the nature of the affected childrens' lives as adults. We can be sure that financial issues will be a constant concern for the families; problems about present funding will merge into uncertainty about long-term financial support unless and until new forms of governmental or private insurance payment are forthcoming. All of these known and unknown problems can and will have important implications for the design of services and for the professionals who bring these services to the children and families in need of them. The medical and social service professions must constantly monitor the changing institutions and attitudes of our society in order to advocate effectively and humanely for the special group of children with long term, complex health care needs. Each of the involved professionals must also offer to these children and their families or caretakers unflagging availability for discussion, consultation and advocacy and a sincere willingness to walk this unfamiliar path with them as their lives unfold.

The movement of children with complex medical problems from acute-care hospitals into home settings is certainly going to increase, driven by many medical and social forces. This significant shift in medical practice and in the expectations of families will continue to generate stress, conflict and uncertainty in the families, the children and the professionals who work with them. Changing social structures and public policies will add to those uncertainties, and new ethical dilemmas will arise. Responsible professionals will be best prepared to meet those needs if they are clearly aware of their own changing values and practices, if they understand the difficulties which the children and families face and honor their concerns and choices, and if they recognize that each decision along the way must be revisited and, if necessary, reshaped as the children's and caretakers' needs evolve.

In a rapidly changing universe, concerned professionals must practice vigilance and adaptability in addition to their particular special skills. The successful placement of medically complex children in home settings is a challenge to traditional concepts of professional authority and to standard ways of practice. Responsive and innovative medical and social service professionals can, through collaboration and persistence, help bring significant numbers of children home whose lives would be otherwise spent in hospitals; with the attendant benefits to the children and happiness and satisfaction to their parents and caretakers.

REFERENCES

Aday, L. A., Aitken, M. J., & Wegener, D. H. (1988). *Pediatric home care: Results of a national evaluation of programs for ventilator assisted children.* Chicago: Pluribus Press.

American Academy of Pediatrics. (1984). Guidelines for home care of infants, children and adolescents with chronic disease. *Pediatrics, 74,* 434–436.

Association for the Care of Children's Health. (1988). *From hospital to home care: An annotated bibliography.* Washington, D.C.: Author.

Association for the Care of Children's Health. (1984). *Home care for children with serious handicapping conditions.* Washington, D.C.: Author.

Corbin, J. M. & Strauss, A. L. (1988). *Unending work and care: Managing chronic illness at home.* San Francisco: Jossey-Bass, Inc.

Department of Health and Human Services (1988). *Report to congress and the secretary by the task force on technology-dependent children (2 vols.).* (HCFA publication No. 88-02171). Washington, D.C.; U.S. Government Printing Office.

Kohrman, A. F. (in press-1990). Psychological issues in pediatric home care. In M. J. Mehlman & S. J. Youngner (Eds.), *Issues in high technology home care: A guide for decision making.* Owings Mills, MD.: National Health Publishing Co.

Office of Technology Assessment (1983). *Technology and Handicapped People.* New York: Springer Publishing Co.

Office of Technology Assessment (1987). *Technology-dependent children: Hospital v. home care—A technical memorandum.* (OTA-TM-H-38). Washington, D.C.: U.S. Government Printing Office.

Schreiner, M. S., Donar, M. E., & Kettrick, R. G. (1987). Pediatric home mechanical ventilation. *Pediatric Clinics of North America, 34,* 47–60.

CHAPTER 2

SPECIALIZED FAMILY FOSTER CARE

JAKE TERPSTRA

INTRODUCTION

It is a strongly held societal value that children are best raised in a family setting. Lieberman (1987) notes that there exists a long history of community, governmental and charitable support for children unable to be cared for adequately by their families. For the past 100 years family foster care has been a major resource in this country for the care of children. Although there has been variation in the needs of children placed in foster care, the range of foster homes has been relatively narrow. Until recently, foster care was perceived to be a short-term arrangement for relatively intact dependent children. While this was not always the case, this was the framework under which the prevailing child welfare philosophy and practice emerged. Although the goal of foster care traditionally has been the reunification of the family, many children were placed for indefinite periods of time in virtual non-legal adoption arrangements. These situations led to the impetus for permanency planning.

At the same time the long-held role of foster parents has been evolving. Historically, foster parents provided physical care and nurturance while agency staff provided case planning, management, counselling and all specialized services. Often, foster parents were minimally involved in these matters as they were expected to serve as substitute parents only. Likewise, minimal training was provided to foster parents as it was assumed they had the requisite parenting skills.

Today, children coming into care have more complex needs and require more specialized care than "traditional" foster homes can provide. Social problems and medical technology are producing children who previously would not have been eligible for foster care. Compounding this problem is the increasing cost of institutional care.

Moreover, the current shortage of foster homes necessitates the need to use existing homes more effectively and to develop alternative resources. There is growing awareness that with training and support, foster parents are able to carry out complex home care tasks with more problematic children than previously believed. Child welfare organizations are now viewing the shift in the foster parents' role as therapeutically desirable. Staff shortages and high turnover have added to the difficulty of making this shift.

THE NEED FOR SPECIALIZED FAMILY FOSTER CARE

An increasing number of children eligible for foster care have extremely serious and complex needs. The reasons for this increase are generally well documented—increased poverty and homelessness, increased drug use on the part of both parents and children, more single parent families, more reliance on medical technology, and an increase in the reported child abuse and neglect. These problems have led to changes in children's services, and in some instances, to the emergence of new types of services. Even though it appears that the growing needs are rapidly overtaking services and resources, there are some encouraging developments; specifically, the increased emphasis on permanency planning for children in foster care. Permanency planning is defined as the process of helping a child to live in a home which offers the hope of establishing lifetime family relationships. This practice has provided a clearer conceptual framework to child welfare than had existed prior to the 1970's. The concepts of permanence were largely institutionalized through Public Law 96-272, the Adoption Assistance and Child Welfare Act of 1980 (Social Security Act, 1935). This law has had a profound effect on child welfare services nationwide and continues to provide a stimulus for the development of new services. Specialized family foster care (SFFC) embodies the concept of permanency planning in the spirit of Public Law 96-272.

SPECIALIZED FAMILY FOSTER CARE

Specialized family foster care (SFFC) has emerged in the last decade as a unique service although antecedents can be found in past practice. This service has given child welfare professionals a new option in their array of resources. In fact, variations of SFFC offer multiple service options that can be used selectively for special needs children. These new resources require commensurate skill on the part of child welfare professionals so they may select options that are directed to the real needs of children and their families.

The needs of children in SFFC may be as varied as those of children in regular family foster care and child care institutions. The decision as to which resources to use is determined by the need of the child, the intensity of the problem and the amount of specialized services required. For children removed from their homes for reasons of parental behavior, rather than child behavior, care in a regular family foster home may be the best resource. On the other end of the continuum are children with severe emotional disturbances, medically complex/fragile children, HIV positive children and severely developmentally disabled children; many of whom receive residential care.

SFFC can serve as an alternative to institutional care and also as a form of after-care following residential services. Many children who otherwise would have to enter far more expensive, and often less conveniently located care, can be served as well in specialized family foster care. This avoids the high cost of institutional care while providing the benefits of a family atmosphere. Many children in institutions, including hospitals, no longer need those services but are able to leave only when an intermediate level of care is available. Thus, SFFC serves as a preventative service, an aftercare service, and as a specific service of first choice.

What is SFFC? Currently, there is a lack of consensus in the child welfare field regarding SFFC's terminology and its essential components. This service may be called professional foster care, treatment foster care, medical foster care, family based treatment, therapeutic foster care or specialized family foster care. A consensus on terms would enhance practice and promote an orderly growth of this service. Consistency in terminology would also make it easier to develop and use payment procedures.

The term "specialized family foster care" is used here because it encompasses the variety of services required by these children. Other terminology is more circumscribed. For example, foster care should be therapeutic even if professional (clinical) therapy is not provided. "Treatment" can occur in almost any setting, including the child's own home or a regular foster home. Specialized family foster care implies that the therapy or treatment emanates from within the foster home. This may be obvious as when a foster parent is selected because of certain professional skills required by the child e.g., nursing, speech

therapy. Generally, however, foster parents do not have these professional skills but may be trained to be used in highly specialized ways
as part of the treatment team. In fact, many agencies have found
their major successes are with persons who are seasoned regular foster
parents recruited for specialized roles. The treatment or therapy emanates from the way the agency and the home work together in concert
toward goals established in the case plan. Treatment goals may be
modified when needs change, with both agency staff, foster parents
and birth parents involved in this process.

As with any field of endeavor, particularly new ones, there invar-
iably is a lack of clarity as to the essence of the service and what
clearly distinguishes it from certain other services. The purpose of
SFFC, and its impact upon children and their families, can be comparable to that of a residential treatment program. A major distinc-
tion however, is that the care occurs in a private family home rather
than in a group care setting with paid staff.

The obvious next question is—how is SFFC distinguished from
regular family foster care? Meisner (personal communication, 1982)
puts the issue into perspective by suggesting the following: ". . . to
understand SFFC one must discard nearly all preconceived ideas
about regular family foster care, thinking instead of the program as
a residential treatment setting and applying that to a family setting."
As Rubenstein, Armentrout, Levin and Harold (1978) stated regarding a Florida SFFC program, "The concept that evolved to meet
the objectives was that of an institution without walls." While there
are specific components common to most SFFC programs the common denominator is the concept of an intensive treatment program
directed specifically to the child's particular needs. Consequently, the
model or format of SFFC, and its overall approach, is more similar
to group residential treatment programs than to regular foster care.
With appropriate training of foster parents and the redevelopment
of existing resources this approach can be emulated by providers of
regular foster care services. In order for regular foster care programs
to develop into actual SFFC *all* of the necessary components must
be incorporated. The failure to do so may well compromise the in-
tegrity and effectiveness of the service.

COMPONENTS OF SFFC

The primary difference between SFFC and other types of foster care
arrangements is the configuration of the service components which

allows for intensive and comprehensive application. The following components are generally found in SFFC:

- Careful selection of foster parents. Foster parents can be recruited for specific skills required to care for a child with a definitive need e.g., nursing, physical therapy or speech therapy. Many successful specialized foster parents can be recruited from existing seasoned regular parents; previous successful experience in caring for children is essential.

- Specialized foster parents' involvement is more intensive than regular foster care. Consequently, one foster parent should be in the home full-time.

- A small number of children should be placed in the home at any one time. The age of the child, type of the problem(s) and the skill level of the foster parent(s) are used in determining the number of children placed in SFFC. Generally, one child but not more than two, are placed in an SFFC.

- Foster parents should be reimbursed or subsidized at higher rates than regular foster parents. In some instances, when agencies pay actual salaries, the foster parents may become agency employees.

- Considerable maturity is required on the part of foster parents. Age and family life cycle are important considerations when recruiting foster parents for SFFC. Generally specialized foster parents are at least in their mid-twenties when recruited.

- Specialized foster parents require intensive training, combining both pre-service and in-service approaches. Much of the training is specifically tailored to the types of problems the parents are likely to encounter. Training also facilitates the use of community resources; especially medical, counselling and educational services.

- Involvement of the agency social work staff is intensive. Decreased case loads (generally no more than 10) allow for more intensive efforts with the child, the foster parents, and if feasible with the birth parents and community resources.

- A comprehensive, flexible array of services such as medical, special education, counselling, support groups, are often essential for children in SFFC.

- Case management by the child welfare staff must be intensive and comprehensive. The case manager must define and orchestrate services for the child, foster family and, if appropriate, the birth family.

- Foster parents, as part of the treatment team, are active participants in case planning and case management.
- Respite care may be an essential component for a successful SFFC. Key factors in successful respite care include a readily accessible facility and making the respite care a pre-planned service. It is also helpful to use the same respite provider(s) so that they understand the needs of the child and can carryout out the goals of the case plan.
- After-care (follow-up) services are essential to a successful SFFC. Although after-care services are generally carried out by social work staff, specialized foster parents may also be trained and/or qualified to carry out this function.
- The administration of an SFFC program is best handled by one person in a multi-service agency. It is critical that the organization support the aims of the program. Clear-cut organizational responsibilities can prevent the dilution of the program's effectiveness.

It is the collective impact of the above components that create the critical mass that sets SFFC apart from regular foster family care. The overarching philosophy which drives the delivery of SFFC is permanency planning. The overall goal of all foster care is for children to return to their own home, or to be placed in a permanent home setting, as soon as possible. Within SFFC the concentration of services should meet the needs of the child, foster family and the birth family; at the same time facilitating the resolution of the permanency goal as quickly as possible. Alternatively, some children may not be able to return home but have made gains sufficient enough that they no longer require SFFC. In those instances the foster home can be adjusted to regular family foster care or can help facilitate the replacement of the child into a more appropriate home. In these instances, the lower regular foster care rate may be an inadvertent disincentive to achieving the goal of permanency planning. If in the course of care it becomes apparent that adoption is the plan of choice the child may be eligible for adoption by the SFFC family. Although these alternatives may represent the loss of a specialized foster care resource for the agency, in the long run it will serve the best interests of the child.

In order to be certain that programs identifying themselves as specialized are indeed that, several states have developed licensing requirements for SFFC. In most states SFFC homes are still licensed as regular foster care. This does not necessarily create problems because an agency can enrich a program above licensing requirements at any time. Therefore, regular foster home licensing requirements do not restrict the development of specialized programs. Specific licensure of SFFC however, does increase the likelihood that specialized components will actually be implemented.

SPECIALIZED FAMILY FOSTER CARE PROGRAMS

Being a relatively new service, SFFC does not have extensive literature. However, some programs have been described in published articles. Some agencies have also developed descriptive program materials. These materials show strong evidence of the diversity, efficacy and economy of these programs. The diversity is rooted in the needs of the child and in the tailoring of program components to meet those needs. Despite this diversity, the program components listed above are incorporated with considerable consistency.

Eagle Village in Hersey, Michigan (Van Den Brink, 1984) is a multi-service agency with 36 emotionally disturbed and delinquent youth in SFFC. With the development of these services the agency was able to serve a more diverse population with virtually the same level of service intensity as carried out in the agency's residential care program; at approximately half the operating cost. Moreover, there were negligible start-up costs. An additional cost benefit was found in the flexibility of the program i.e., as needs or resources shifted there were no empty beds or costly buildings to be maintained. There were also program advantages in that the large number of SFFC homes developed enabled careful matching of children with care providers. This program found that birth parents were more willing to be involved in the informal SFFC setting and that children were able to return home in seven to eight months due to the intense family counselling provided.

SFFC was developed by the Children's Crisis Center, Jacksonville, Florida to prevent extended hospital stays for children with complex medical conditions (e.g., ventilator dependent children, tracheotomy care, burn care, tube feeding) when the child's parents were unable to cope (Davis, Foster & Whitworth, 1986). The aims of the program were to reduce extended hospitalization, and improve functioniong of birth families, by using families in which one foster parent was a registered nurse. Not only were children returned to their families much sooner but there were significant cost savings associated with the reduced need for hospital care. Similarly, Arcari & Betman (1986) showed that specialized foster care lends itself to the care of deaf children.

A program funded by the Children's Bureau of the United States Department of Health and Human Services for children with complex medical conditions was developed by the Children's Home and Aid Society of Illinois and La Rabida Children's Hospital (Yost, Hochstadt & Charles, 1988). This intense program placed seven medically complex children in SFFC during the initial two years of the program. One child was returned to his mother and another to relatives while five were cared for in SFFC. The project made it possible for children to live in families, including their own, rather remaining in hospitals for extended periods. Cost savings were as much as $14,000 per month per child (Hochstadt & Yost, 1989).

The Massachusetts Department of Social Services developed a project called Parents and Children together (Matava, 1986) which served about 100 children in 65 family homes. Children ranged from troubled pregnant girls to developmentally delayed infants. This program showed that intense efforts make it possible to meet a wide range of needs, with a high incidence of return to birth families.

Presley Ridge School in Pittsburgh (Meadowcroft, Trout & Luster, 1985) served over 100 children from 1981 to 1985. Children's ages ranged from 4 to 18 years, with a majority between 13 and 17 years. Aggressive behavior and hyperactivity were prevalent. In spite of this, 82% of the youngsters were successfully treated as measured by the stringent criteria developed by this agency.

A demonstration/research project in Oregon (Chamberlain, 1990), also funded by the Children's Bureau of the United States Department of Health and Human Services, placed sixteen 12–18-year-old delinquent youths in SFFC. The project was carried out between January, 1984 and April, 1986. It included a control group of 16 youths who were matched by age, sex and date of commitment. Seventy-five percent of each group had been incarcerated the previous year. During the first year 6 (38%) of the SFFC group were reinstitutionalized, while 14 (88%) of the control group were reinstitutionalized. While the difference was less striking during the second year, the reincarceration rate for the SFFC group for the two year period was 50%, while the rate for the control group was 94%. Other evidence of the efficacy of SFFC is the fact that the more days these children spent in SFFC the less time they spent incarcerated. There was no such positive correlation for the control (non-SFFC) group.

These brief descriptions of a few of the many programs throughout the country demonstrate the broad range of needs that can be met by SFFC. These studies consistently indicate the need for strong commitment by both the agency and the SFFC homes in order for a viable program to evolve. The program components, noted above, with some variation, are present in each of the above programs. These programs demonstrate that strong, knowledgeable commitment pays off. The benefit to children and their families, and the cost savings, when compared with traditional alternatives, are striking.

ETHICAL AND OTHER CONSIDERATIONS

When resources are scarce they may have to be rationed or allocated very judiciously to meet the individual needs of children. While SFFC programs are generally less costly than residential care they are still more costly than traditional foster care. Many agencies have found that the costs of SFFC are approximately half that of residential care. Nevertheless, SFFC may cost as much as $9,000 a month when professional nursing services are needed 16 hours a day. When compared with the $23,000 a month cost for hospital care a significant savings is realized. However, even the lower cost of SFFC can be devastating to the budgets of some agencies and such outlays must be made selectively. Most SFFC programs have demonstrated that the amount of time needed to accomplish case goals are as short as, or shorter than, residential care. Re-entry and residivism rates are also lower. Consequently, it is incumbent upon agency staff to know each child and the resources available so as to make judicious decisions regarding resource allocation. At a minimum, agencies must consider all of the implications surrounding resource allocation issues, i.e., human and fiscal. Agency staff should have strong support for comprehensive staff training to prepare them to adequately evaluate the needs of children and to assess the availability of resources. When the placement of children is being considered there are only two overriding questions: what is best for the child and the family? And what is possible?

CONCLUSION

Currently, SFFC offers a valuable new addition to the spectrum of child welfare services needed to care for the ever growing population of needy children with complex needs entering foster care. It is important that a balance be struck between more traditional foster care services and innovative approaches. Given current trends, it is conceivable that with time SFFC will develop to the point that it will be the primary resource for substitute care. An organization, called the Family Based Treatment Association, was recently created to develop a network of specialized home programs and to focus professional attention on this growing new service. This association also holds national conferences, and publishes literature on SFFC. These activities should contribute to the development of clearer concepts of SFFC including a nationwide awareness of both its strengths and limitations.

REFERENCES

Acari, T. M. & Bertram, B. G. (1986). The deaf child in foster care. *Children Today*.

Chamberlain, P., & Weinrott, M. (1990). Specialized foster care: Treating seriously emotionally disturbed children. *Children Today*. January-February, 204–227.

Davis, A. B., Foster, P. H. & Whitworth, J. M. (1984). Medical foster family care—a cost effective solution to a community problem. *Child Welfare, 63*, 341–349.

Hochstadt, N. J. & Yost, D. M. (1989). The health care—child welfare partnership: Transitioning medically complex children to the community. *Children's Health Care, 18*, 4–11.

Lieberman, F. (1987). Clinical practice and the special issues of foster care. *Child and Adolescent Social Work, 4*, 3–9.

Matawa, M. A. (1986). *A specialized foster care project*. (Available from [Massachusetts Department of Social Services, Boston, MA]).

Meadowcroft, P., Trout, B. A., & Clark, L. W. (1985). *Journal of Clinical Psychology, 4*, 220–228.

Rubenstein, J. S., Armentrout, J. A., Levin, S. & Harold, D. (1978). The parent-therapist program: Alternative care for emotionally disturbed children. *American Journal of Orthopsychiatry, 48*, 654–662.

Social Security Act of 1935, 602, U.S.C. 402 Title IV (1980).

Van Den Brink (1984). Expanding the options. *Children Today*, March-April, 32–35.

Yost, D. M., Hochstadt, N. J. & Charles P. (1988). Medical foster care, achieving permanency for seriously ill children. *Children Today*, 5, 22–26.

92-61

Section II
Medical Overview

CHAPTER 3

THE MEDICAL CARE OF CHILDREN WITH COMPLEX HOME HEALTH CARE NEEDS: AN OVERVIEW FOR CARETAKERS

PAULA KIENBERGER JAUDES

INTRODUCTION

Long before the advent of hospitals, founded in the 18th century as institutions of care for the sick, home was the place children received their health care. Historically, physicians cared for the sick in the patient's own home with mothers and family members performing the nursing and medical tasks. It is ironic that home care has come back into fashion as clinical and technological achievements have exploded. Home care brings with it both a change of locus and focus of care for many seriously ill, chronically ill and technology-dependent children who are in hospitals. Today, home care as an alternative to institutional care is one of the most rapidly growing fields of medicine; with no signs of slowing down in the twenty-first century.

Cost is one of the motivating factors behind the increase in home care. Originally, home care was thought to be less expensive than hospital/institutional care. But this is not always the case. Home care may potentially be less expensive but not by much when one factors in the cost of family-supplied care, parental loss of employment, food, educational charges, home renovations, etc. Therefore, home care should be thought of less as a cost-saving measure than as an attempt to normalize the life of a child within a family and community setting.

The goal of home care is the provision of health care within a nurturing home environment that maximizes the capabilities of the child and minimizes the effects of the disability. However, home care is not for everyone. The American Academy of Pediatrics Ad Hoc

29

Task Force on Home Care of the Chronically Ill Infants and Children (1984) has set criteria which must be met by the patient, the family and the community before discharge planning can begin. For the child, the medical condition must be stable with back up and emergency care in place. For the caretakers, they must be able to perform all the nursing and medical tasks necessary for the child in the home and these capabilities must be demonstrated in the hospital setting before discharge. For many of the medical conditions, two family members need to be trained and capable of caring for the child. They must be able to perform all the nursing and medical tasks necessary for the child to be safely cared for in the home. For some families, the interest or capabilities may not be present. In those cases, alternative family members or foster parents may fill the role of caretaker in the home. In the community, a local physician must be available to provide primary care for the child. The community must also be able to provide educational services, health care providers, and requisite equipment.

Once these criteria are met, discharge planning is best conducted by an interdisciplinary team to provide a comprehensive, coordinated care plan. This plan should identify a case coordinator, a defined back-up system for medical emergencies and family access to a telephone. It is important that the plan be well thought out and flexible enough for adjustments to be made when needed. Of paramount importance is the presence of a primary care physician, the appropriate developmental, educational, rehabilitative services, some mechanism for providing continuing social and emotional support for the child and the family, appropriate respite care as needed, hospital care, and if necessary, alternative long-term placement. Parents and alternative caretakers must be allowed guilt-free renegotiation about their decision for home care during, and even after discharge. At any time, and for whatever reason, parents can and may change their minds about caring for the child in the home. Alternative plans should be in place to comply with this change of mind. Parents should not feel trapped into taking care of the child in the home (Stein & Jessop, 1984).

It must be remembered that some children with relatively stable medical conditions will always be at risk for a major catastrophe no matter where they are, even in the hospital. Two purposes of the discharge plan are to make the home environment as safe a place as possible and to train the caretakers thoroughly and knowledgeably in the care of the child. However, given the best of training and intentions, problems may still occur. Caretakers and health care workers need to understand and accept the fact that these children may always be at risk for emergency situations.

The next section contains brief general descriptions of the most common pediatric medical problems treated in the home and the community. Specific details are given concerning the activities performed, and the equipment needed, by home caregivers. A more comprehensive description of the medical issues can be found by referring to the references at the end of each section. For further description of the generic issues of home health care discussed in this introduction, refer to the following references: Association for the Care of Children's Health (1984); Association for the Care of Children's Health (1988); Committee on Children with Disabilities (1986); American Academy of Pediatrics, Ad Hoc Task Force on Home Care of Chronically Ill Infants and Children (1984); Halpern (1986); and Stein and Jessop (1984).

NUTRITIONAL PROBLEMS

There are multiple reasons why a child cannot take food by mouth, including congenital anomalies of the oral pharyngeal area, congenital anomalies of the gastrointestinal tract, short bowel syndrome, intractable diarrhea, inflammatory bowel disease, cancer, inborn errors of metabolism, increased metabolic needs, severe cerebral palsy, uncoordinated swallowing, heart-lung disease, kidney failure, liver dysfunction, oral hypersensitivity, and central nervous system disorders. Also, there are some children who can feed by mouth but who cannot take in enough calories to meet their caloric needs. Other than by mouth, two different routes can provide nutritional support for the child: enteral and parenteral. Which route is implemented depends on the nature of the child's medical condition.

Enteral nutrition involves placing nutrition directly into the gastrointestinal tract by means of a tube: either a nasogastric tube (N/G), or a gastrostomy tube (G-tube). If a child's gastrointestinal tract can absorb nutrients then enteral feeding can be done. If a child is expected to need enteral nutrition for only a short time, then a N/G tube is usually the choice. However, if a child is not expected to be able to feed for six months or more, then surgery is usually performed to place a tube in the stomach (G-tube).

Caretakers must know how to care for the skin around the tube, as well as how to anchor, change and identify problems with the tube.

Initially, caretakers may be reluctant and afraid to replace tubes, but with education and experience they adapt very well. The equipment and materials needed are minimal and include: tubes, feeding bags, IV pole, syringes, and dressing care materials. The specific nutrition required is based on the age and the medical condition of the child. Usually commercially prepared formula or home prepared blender-ized food is utilized. The number and times of feeding depends on the exact medical needs and the absorptive capabilities of the child's gastrointestinal tract.

Total parenteral nutrition (TPN) provides nutrition to patients whose medical illness prevents the use of the gastrointestinal tract to obtain adequate nutrition. Nutrients are supplied directly into the blood-stream by a central line catheter, usually placed in the large superior vena cava vein located on the right side of the chest. Proper care of the central line is extremely important to prevent blockage of the line or infection of the child from the line causing rehospitalization and additional surgery. Parenteral nutrition consists of two solutions: (1) hyperalimentation—a clear/yellow solution which comes in a plas-tic bag containing amino acids (proteins), dextrose (sugar), minerals, and vitamins; and (2) lipids—a milky white solution which comes in a small glass bottle contains fat. The solutions are usually made by the pharmaceutical company or hospital pharmacy and delivered to the home. Caretakes are instructed in the amounts, frequencies and solution(s) to use. A child on home parenteral nutrition is usually so stable that the composition of the solutions only change weekly. Most children receive parental nutrition infusions 10–16 hours a day. Blood is drawn in the home by home health agency personnel once a week to monitor the electrolytes and nutrients of the child.

Caretakers must be trained in proper techniques for central line catheter care, how to administer parenteral nutrition and maintain the equipment. Equipment and materials needed include: electric pumps requiring grounded electrical outlets, tubing, clamps, dressing care materials, thermometer, weighing scale and urine testing sup-plies. For further information concerning the nutritional issues of home health care discussed in this section, see: Alltop (1988); Paarl-berg & Balint (1985); Gullate (1989); Barber (1984); and Rivard (1989).

PULMONARY PROBLEMS

There are many different pulmonary problems which can affect chil-dren. The most common of the pulmonary illnesses and technology-dependent conditions which may require home health care include asthma, bronchopulmonary dysplasia, cystic fibrosis, tracheostomy and ventilator dependency.

Asthma

Asthma is the most common chronic disease of childhood with approximately 10–12% of all children having this disease at some time in their lives. Asthma is an airway disease manifested by recurrent reversible airway obstruction. The obstruction or narrowing of the breathing tubes (bronchi), is caused by spasm of the bronchial smooth muscles, production of tenacious mucous secretions and swelling of the lining of the bronchiols. Triggers of this obstruction may be manyfold and include allergens, exercise, emotions, weather, infection, chemicals and irritants. Asthma can cause symptoms of coughing, wheezing, shortness of breath, difficulty in breathing, decreased level of activity, and rarely cyanosis, lethargy, coma and death.

Medical care involves a two pronged approach involving (1) taking medication to prevent or reverse the airway obstruction (2) controlling the environment to remove the triggers of the obstruction. When allergens are the trigger for asthma, then removal of the offending allergens is essential. Common allergens include animal dander, house dust mite (found in rugs, stuffed animals, upholstered furniture, and mattresses) molds, and occasionally foods. There are numerous medications in a wide variety of forms available for the control of asthma. The five basic groups of medications used in the treatment of asthma are theophylline, beta adrenergics, anticholinergics, cromolyn sodium, and steroids.

Theophylline is the medication most commonly used and is thought to act as a relaxant of the bronchial muscle. This medication is given by mouth every six, eight, or twelve hours depending on the preparation. Beta agonist medications are also bronchodilators and may be given by mouth, inhalation or injection. Inhalation is the fastest, most direct, and effective route for the medication to reach the lung directly. Inhalation can be accomplished by using either a handheld nebulizer or metered dose inhalers (MDI). The medication and a diluent, usually normal saline solution, are added to the nebulizer, while a small air compressor unit powers the nebulizer creating a mist solution which the child inhales. The mist is delivered to the child via a mouth piece, a mask, or a tracheostomy collar. This mode of delivery does not require the participation of the child. MDIs are small cannisters containing medication and a propellant. When activated, they deliver an aerosol of medication which is inhaled by the patient. Its use however, requires a degree of participation by the patient and therefore, are only used by older children. MDIs can be used with a spacer device which enhances the delivery of medication. Anticholinergics act by inhibiting reflex bronchoconstriction. This medication is given by inhalation. Cromolyn sodium is a medication used to prevent wheezing attacks. Cromolyn sodium is also administered by inhalation. Steroids are thought to reduce bronchial inflammation and edema. This group of medications is used in short courses to end an attack, in serious attacks of asthma, or as longterm therapy for difficult to control asthma. Their long-term use is limited because of the numerous adverse side effects. Steroids can be given by mouth or MDI. A child with difficult to control asthma may be given one, two or all types of medication by mouth and/or inhalation.

Caretakers should be taught to recognize signs and symptoms of an asthma attack, to control an asthma attack in the home by administrating medicine and inhalation therapies, and knowing when to take the child to seek additional medical help. For further description of asthma, see: Lucas, Golish, Sleeper and O'Ryan (1988); Goldenhersh and Rachelefsky (1989); Rachelefsky (1984); and Harper and Strunk (1981).

Bronchopulmonary Dysplasia

Bronchopulmonary Dysplasia (BPD) is a chronic lung disease of infancy that affects primarily premature babies. Most of these infants required mechanical ventilation in the nursery for a period of time. The disease results from lung damage from several causes which leads to abnormal growth of both the bronchial tree and the lung tissue causing the lung to work less effectively. Children with BPD breathe faster and with more effort than normal children; they may need oxygen. Children with BPD also have some of the same signs and symptoms as children with asthma.

Many children with BPD need oxygen therapy. The oxygen can be administered to the child in the home by the method of nasal cannula or tracheostomy collar. There are three systems commonly used in the home to deliver oxygen: high-pressure cylinders, liquid oxygen systems, and oxygen concentrators. High-pressure gas cylinders come in several sizes and must be stablized in an area where they cannot be knocked over. Oxygen can be compressed into a liquid so tanks can be small and easily portable. Oxygen concentrators are machines, run by electricity, that separate oxygen from other gases in the atmosphere. This system is more commonly used in rural areas not served by oxygen supply companies, or when large amounts of oxygen are needed. Backup oxygen cylinders are required in case of electrical failure. All tanks have either a flow meter or a restrictor that adjusts the amount of oxygen flow to the patient. Humidity is important to keep the respiratory tract moist and to decrease dryness of the nose. A bottle of water can be attached to the oxygen system to provide humidity. Routine measurement of the blood oxygen saturation level is done by application of a probe to the child's finger, ear or toe. The oxygen flow can be then adjusted to provide optimal blood oxygen saturation.

Chest physical therapy (CPT) is a mechanical technique to facilitate the removal of bronchial secretions. The chest is tapped firmly by hand, a rubber percussor, or an electric percussor while the child's body is placed in different positions. This helps secretions to drain from a more peripheral area in the lung to larger airways where the secretions can be coughed up. For some children, secretions may need to be removed by a suctioning machine using suction catheters and sterile saline to loosen the tenacious secretions.

Many of the same medications used to treat asthma are also used in the treatment of BPD: theophylline, beta adrenergics, anticholinergics, steroids, and cromolyn sodium. These medications can be given by mouth and/or home nebulizer. A nebulizer is a machine which converts a liquid (medicine) to a fine spray. Diuretics are also utilized because they decrease the amount of fluid in the lungs. This helps the lung work more effectively. Certain diuretics can cause a loss of potassium in the urine; their use necessitates oral supplementation with potassium salts.

In order for children with BPD to get better, they need to grow new lung tissue around the scarred areas. Nutrition is extremely important not only for the growth of these sick children but expecially for the growth of new lung tissue. Children with respiratory difficulties utilize more calories because of the increased work of breathing; thus, children may require supplemental nutrients and high calorie foods.

Caretakers should be taught to monitor oxygen therapy; perform chest physical therapy; administer medications; recognize adequate nutrition and methods of feeding; how to help the infant develop and learn; monitor apnea; perform CPR; assess the child and know when to get medical help and emergency medical care; and to cope with the demands of care. For further explanations of bronchopulmonary dysplasia, see: Perry and Hayes (1988); and Hanson (1987).

Cystic Fibrosis

Cystic Fibrosis (CF) is an inherited disorder affecting the sodium and chloride transport across epithelial (membrane) surfaces. The mucous membranes produce abnormally thick secretions. The two major problems for these patients are pancreatic digestive enzyme blockage and pulmonary disease caused by these thick secretions. The pancreatic ducts become blocked and glued by the abnormal viscous secretions of the pancreas so that digestive pancreatic enzymes are unable to reach the food to digest it. The lung also has abnormal thick viscous mucous resulting in progressive pulmonary infections. Cystic fibrosis is in most cases, a slow, progressive disease with an average life expectancy of twenty years.

Treatment of the clinical manifestations of pancreatic duct blockage consists mainly in replacement of the pancreatic enzymes by taking medicine in the form of a pill(s) at meal times. Vitamins are also indicated. Many children with CF have poor weight gain or weight loss and may need supplemental calories. This may be accomplished by N/G feedings at night or TPN (as discussed earlier). Treatment of the pulmonary problems is more difficult. Depending on the medical center, home treatment by the administrations of antibiotics to combat pulmonary infections may be given. These antibiotics may be administered by mouth, intravenously or nebulized. Chest physical therapy, usually with vibration and/or clapping with postural drainage, should be done frequently each day for most of these children; this aids in mobilizing secretions. Some children may be on bronchodilators, mucolytic agents, antimicrobial agents (as discussed earlier) or antiflammatory agents (corticosteroids or cromolyn) which may all be given by nebulization. The bronchodilators and mucolytic agents are given prior to chest physiotherapy.

Caretakers may need to be taught skills in administration of medicines; care and placement of N/G tube; nutrition; TPN; chest physical therapy; and administration of nebulizations. Both child and caretaker may need psychosocial counseling concerning caring for, and living with, this chronic illness. For further description of cystic fibrosis, see: Stern (1989); Donati, Guenette and Auerbach (1987); Wheeler and Colten (1988); and Cunningham and Taussig (1989).

Tracheostomy

Tracheostomy tubes are placed in children for a number of conditions including vocal cord paralysis, subglottic stenosis, croup, BPD or obstructive apnea. Tracheostomy refers to an opening in the neck from skin to the trachea (windpipe) in which a tube is placed. The purpose of the tube is to establish and maintain an open airway from the lungs to the outside, circumventing the obstructed area above the tracheostomy. Sizes and types of tubes vary. Children breathe air directly from the tracheostomy into the lungs, bypassing the vocal cords, the nose and the mouth. Because of this, two important functions are lost, requiring supplemental measures. Normally, the nose and mouth humidify the air which is breathed, keeping the secretions in the lungs loose and easily movable. A child with a tracheostomy will need a humidifier to deliver the humidity directly to the tracheostomy by means of a tracheostomy collar. Additionally, plastic heat and moisture exchangers (HME) are attached to the tracheostomy tube to trap the moisture as the child breathes out and then humidify the air as the child breathes in. Speech is the second lost function. Vocalization, ordinarily accomplished by air passing over the vocal cords with the mouth forming words, becomes for many of these children an impossible task. As a result, communication becomes problematic and the children and families may need to learn sign language as a means of communication. There are now available speaking valves which attach to the tracheostomy which allows for some children with tracheostomies to talk.

Since the tracheostomy is the only open airway the child has, diligence in keeping it open is essential. Changing the tracheostomy tube is a two person procedure. Suctioning of mucous from the trachea must be performed as needed to clear the trachea of secretions to make it easier for the child to breathe. In times of respiratory illness, suctioning may be needed more often. A child with a tracheostomy must be watched at all times and when the child is sleeping, an apnea monitor must be attached to alert the caretaker of breathing problems or plugged tracheostomy. At least two caretakers must be trained in the care of tracheostomy because of the potential life threatening nature of this condition.

The two **caretakers** need to be trained in the signs and symptoms of respiratory distress; how to suction by aseptic technique; how to change the tracheostomy tube; care and cleaning of the tracheostomy tube; equipment care; sign language; cardiopulmonary resuscitation; and what to do in an emergency. Necessary home equipment includes portable battery-operated suction machine, connecting tube for the suction, apnea monitor and leads, hand resuscitator bag, sterile normal saline, vinegar, twill tape, pipe cleaners, tracheostomy dressing, hydrogen peroxide, tracheostomy tubes, humidifier, as well as a telephone with emergency phone numbers available. For further description of the care of tracheostomies discussed in this section, see: Okamoto, Fee, Boles, Calcaterra, Dobie and Steadmen (1977); Foster and Hoskins (1981); Mapp (1988) and Hazinski (1986).

Ventilator Dependency

Ventilator dependency for children may be caused by major lung, muscle or neurological problems preventing the child from adequately breathing to maintain life. All children who are long-term ventilator dependent will have a tracheostomy. The child is attached to the ventilator by the tracheostomy. Children are sent home on a time-cycled, volume limited ventilator.

Not all children who are chronically ventilator dependent become candidates for home care. Those who do must meet the necessary criteria which include: medical stability with no acute pulmonary abnormalities; competent trainable family to care for the child; dependable health professionals in-home support staff; home environment conducive to the patient; and electrical facilities adequate to safely operate all equipment.

The **caretakers** need to be educated in the management of the ventilator, suctioning, tracheal opening and tube care, signs of pulmonary infection, and vital signs and cardiopulmonary resuscitation. Equipment and supplies needed in the home include primary and backup ventilators, suction equipment, tracheostomy supplies, oxygen source, supplemental airway humidity, bed, and a telephone with emergency phone number listings. Psychological support for the child and the caretakers is essential. Respite and periodic follow-up need to be arranged before discharge. A backup plan should also be in place if home care fails. For further information on ventilators and home mechanical ventilation, refer to: O'Ryan and Burns (1984);

Schreiner, Donar and Kettrick (1987); Burr, Guyer, Todres, Abrahams and Chiodo (1983); Fischer (1985); O'Donohue, Giovannoni, Keens and Plummer (1986); and Lucas, Golish, Sleeper and O'Ryan (1988).

NEUROMUSCULAR PROBLEMS

There are many different neurological and muscular problems which can afflict children. Some of the disorders that may require home health intervention include apnea, developmental delay, cerebral palsy, spina bifida and seizures.

Apnea

Apnea is the cessation of breathing for twenty seconds or longer, or for shorter episodes associated with pallor, cyanosis or decreased heart rate. There are numerous causes of apnea including immaturity of the neurological system, metabolic disorders, cardiac problems, acute infections such as sepsis, gastroesophageal reflux, seizures, upper airway obstruction or central nervous system dysfunction. Infantile apnea is thought to result from an immature neurological system. Although the cause(s) of Sudden Infant Death Syndrome (SIDS) is unknown, some of the causes of infantile apneas are thought to represent the same disease process as SIDS. Thus, children with infantile apnea may be at high risk for sudden death. Substantial distress in the home can result from caring for these children due to the inherent problems of monitoring and the risk of death.

Once the diagnosis has been made by the physician, the methods of treatment include medication and/or home monitoring of the child. The medication generally prescribed is theophylline which must be given every six to eight hours. The apnea monitor is a machine which continuously checks the respiratory rate of the infant and sounds an alarm if breathing stops for more than 20 seconds. There are several types of machines all requiring grounded outlets. The two most common methods of monitoring respiratory rate used by the machines are by the electrode belt or skin electrodes. The belt wraps around an infant's chest with the electrodes attached to the belt. The skin electrodes are adhesive and are directly attached to the skin. Telephone installation and community emergency support plans need to be prearranged before the child goes home. Children with infantile apnea usually grow out of this problem and only need to be monitored until six to twelve months of age.

The **caretakers** are trained to identify an apneic spell, to respond to an episode, and to give cardiopulmonary resuscitation in case the child does not respond to stimulation. Equipment needs include apnea monitor, attachable electrodes and telephone. For further information about apnea, see: Brown (1984); Ariagno and Glotzbach (1987); McBride (1984) Garber and Balas-Stevens (1984); Ariango (1984); Norris-Berkemeyer and Hutchins (1986); and Wasserman (1984).

Developmental Delay

Developmental delay (DD) is a term used to describe children who are behind in their attainment of developmental milestones. The term developmental delay is usually applied to children up to five years of age. There are many tests to measure the child's developmental milestones. Measurements includes parents' report and observations. Milestones are assessed in a variety of areas, usually including gross motor, fine motor, oral motor, speech and language, cognition and social development. A child may be delayed in one or more of these areas. Developmental delay is considered when the child exhibits a 25% delay in one area, a 20% delay in two or more areas or a 20% delay in one area with a high probability that the delay will continue or become worse due to environmental risks. Parents of children ages 0 to 3 years who have developmental delay are often referred to an early intervention program. Early intervention programs work with parents to facilitate the child's developmental progress. For further information about developmental delay and handicaps, see: Batshaw and Perret (1987); and Russman (1983).

Cerebral Palsy

Cerebral palsy (CP) is a neuromusular disorder of movement and posture due to brain damage of the motor cortex. The classification of CP is based on the type of movement such as spastic (tight), athetoid (moving), rigid (lead pipe), ataxic (wobbly), atonic (floppy), or mixed (several types). Classification is also based on the part of the body affected such as one limb (monoplegia), both limbs on the same side of body (hemiplegia), lower limbs more than upper limbs (diplegia), three limbs (triplegia), and all four limbs and trunk (quadriplegia). The diagnosis of cerebral palsy is based on an assessment of developmental risk factors, and a complete neurological examination assessing muscle tone, deep tendon reflexes and primitive reflexes. Some of the frequently associated disorders and complications of cerebral palsy include mental retardation, seizures, learning disabilities, visual and hearing impairment, and skeletal deformities. Abnormal movement and posturing may be found in the first year of life but the definitive diagnosis of cerebral palsy is usually not made until two years of age. Signs of gross motor problems or developmental delay are usually picked up much earlier. There are multiple causes of CP ranging from genetic to factors affecting conception, prenatal problems, perinatal problems, to head trauma and central nervous system infection postnatally.

Since CP can be a complex disorder affecting many areas of functioning, management should be directed by an interdisciplinary group composed of an orthopedic surgeon, neurologist, pediatrician, physical therapist, occupational therapist, speech therapist, social worker, orthotics specialist, psychologist and vocational counselor. Unfortunately, there is no conclusive evidence to indicate that specific intervention strategies affect the natural course of this motor disorder. Therefore, there are many different opinions about the type, the timing and the amount of interventions that are necessary to manage this gross motor problem. This indecision can confuse and frustrate caretakers who hear differing opinions from professionals. It is generally accepted, that early intervention programs improve the well being of the child and the caretakers. Also, physical therapy helps prevent contractures and may help maximize the level of functional ability. Bracing and/or surgery may be needed to control abnormal posture, for functional improvement and for prevention and correction of deformities. Muscle relaxants may be used to help decrease spasticity.

Caretakers may need to take the young child to physical and/or occupational therapy sessions on a weekly or semiweekly basis or receive therapy in the home. School age children from three years on, often receive these therapies in school. Caretakers should be taught the motor intervention strategies in order to perform these interventions in the home. Depending on associated problems, a caretaker may need to be trained in other areas needing intervention including feeding, nutrition, speech, seizure control, hearing and visual difficulties, and mental retardation. Caretakers may need to take the child to multiple professionals at several locations. This often proves to be very taxing on the caretakers. Equipment needs for gross motor problems may include leg or back braces, splints, walker, canes, wheelchair, adaptive equipment for feeding, bathing, sitting, a lift, a ramp or an elevator. For further description of cerebral palsy, see: Taft (1984); and Batshaw and Perret (1986).

Spina Bifida

Spina Bifida or myelomeningocele is an open defect in the bony spinal canal on the back (spine) resulting in an outpouching of the spinal cord. This defect is an outcome of abnormal fetal development. The etiology of this disorder is unknown but felt to be multifactorial. The herniation of the spinal cord results in a damage to the cord and, as a result, impairs the functioning of all the nerve and muscle areas controlled at and below the lesion of the spinal cord (Cervical, Thoracic, or Lumbar spinal cord levels). The extent of problems for the child depends at which level the bony defect occurs. The disabilities resulting from the spinal cord damage include flaccid paralysis (very weak or no muscle function) of the lower extremities and trunk, muscle imbalance in the lower extremities resulting in bony deformities such as scoliosis and club feet, loss of sensation, and often, bladder paralysis, bowel paralysis, and hydrocephalus. Bladder paralysis means that the child cannot control the emptying of the bladder and thus is incontinent of urine. Bowel paralysis means that the child cannot control the emptying of the intestines and thus is incontinent of stools. Hydrocephalus is the build up of fluid in the brain as a result of blockage of the circulation of the spinal fluid. This increased fluid produces pressure which compresses the brain and nerve cells. Untreated hydrocephalus can cause mental retardation.

Treatment of spina bifida includes closure of the defect on the back shortly after birth. Motor problems are managed by physical and occupational therapists. The goal of treatment is to strengthen muscles. They also assist in teaching the parents and the child to apply adaptive braces and equipment for functioning. The ability of the child to walk depends on the level of lesion of the spinal cord affected; the higher the lesion the less likely the child will walk. Conversely, the lower the lesion the more likely the child will walk. Occasionally, children may need to undergo orthopedic surgeries to correct bony deformities. Bladder emptying is commonly accomplished by self-insertion of a rubber tube through the urethra into the bladder several times a day. Children with abnormal bladder functions are more prone to bladder infections. If the bladder is not emptied, urine will stagnate and an infection will develop. Medications are often used to help keep a child dry between catheterizations. Bowel emptying is accomplished by nutritional and medical interventions designed for emptying of the bowel in the toilet. If the bowel is not emptied, blockage of the intestines can happen. Toileting skills are important activities of daily living which need to be mastered. Hydrocephalus is treated by the insertion of a plastic tube from the brain to the heart (ventriculo-atrial shunt, VA shunt) or to the abdomen (ventriculo-peritoneal shunt, VP shunt) which drains the fluid and prevents further blockage of the fluid. Many of these children will have learning disabilities. Psycho-education testing is recommended to develop an individual educational program to be instituted at school.

Caretakers need to be trained to perform range of motion and strengthening exercises as well as the use of braces and adaptive equipment. They need to be taught the signs and symptoms of a urinary infection and how to perform intermittent catheterizations of the bladder with a clean technique. Education concerning nutritional issues is important not only for bowel management but also to prevent obesity. For bowel problems, medication regimens need to be learned in addition to technique of giving enemas. Caretakers need to know how to care for desensitized skin including pressure relief and care of skin breakdown. Caretakers must also know the signs and symptoms of shunt obstruction and what to do if there is suspicion of an obstruction. Also, caretakers must gain an understanding of such child related issues as self esteem, body image, sexuality, and dealing with disability. Caretakers may need to advocate for the child to have appropriate psycho-educational testing performed in the school and to obtain an education in the appropriate, and least restrictive environment. Equipment needs include adaptive equipment such as parapodium, caster cart, standing brace, wheelchair, and leg braces, urinary catheters, disposable diapers, training pants, sheepskins, special mattress, and cushions. For further information on spina bifida, see: Bleck and Nagel (1982).

Seizures

Seizures (convulsions) are caused by an abnormal excessive electrical discharge of an area of the brain which may cause alteration of con-

sciousness, involuntary movements and/or abnormal sensory phe-
nomena. Epilepsy is the term to describe repeated seizures. The most
common types of seizures include grand mal, petit mal, atonic, or
partial seizures. Grand mal seizures occur when a child loses consciousness, becomes rigid and then develops rhythmic jerking. This
type of seizure is associated with incontinence, usually last less than
five minutes and is followed by a deep sleep. Petit mal are absence
seizures in which a child stares vacantly into space, blinks, and mo-
mentarily loses consciousness. This is a short seizure, usually lasting
less than 10 seconds. There is no loss of motor control. Atonic seizures
are characterized by an involuntary sudden loss in muscle control and
the child usually falls to the floor. The seizure lasts a few seconds
and the child recovers quickly. Partial seizures are localized to one
part of the brain and, depending on that area, manifest outward signs,
such as a single arm jerking or lip smacking.

The diagnosis of seizures is based on clinical history. Electroen-
cephalogram (EEG) measures the electrical activity of the brain and
can record most abnormal electrical activity. Children are given an-
ticonvulsant medicine to suppress these abnormal electrical dis-
charges.

Caretakers need to be educated in the identification of a seizure;
what to do in the event of a seizure such as protecting the child from
hurting himself/herself; the importance of not leaving the child un-
attended in potentially life threatening environments where the child
might have a seizure (bathtub, swimming pool); how to give anti-
convulsants; what side effects of the medicine to look for, and when
to take the child to the hospital. No special equipment is needed.
For further information on seizures, see: Batshaw and Perret (1987).

KIDNEY PROBLEMS

One of the major functions of the kidneys is to filter the blood,
removing waste and toxins. When the child's kidneys fail to perform
this vital function, there are artificial ways to filter out these wastes
by direct removal from the blood (hemodialysis) or indirect removal
from the lining of the abdomen (peritoneal dialysis). The most common type of dialysis used in the home is peritoneal.

Peritoneal dialysis is performed by introducing one to three liters
of sugar containing salt solution into the peritoneal (abdominal) cavity. By diffusion and ultrafiltration, waste materials move from the

blood into the dialysate solution in the cavity. The solution is then drained from the peritoneal cavity, thus removing the waste and excess water. There are several types of schedules for peritoneal dialysis; the two most common are continuous ambulatory peritoneal dialysis (CAPD) and continuous cycler-assisted peritoneal dialysis (CCPD). For CAPD, the dialysate is always present in the abdomen and is exchanged 4–5 times a day. For CCPD, dialysis begins at night when the patient connects a cycler machine. The machine periodically exchanges the dialysate solution 3–5 times during the night. In the morning, a fresh dialysis solution is left in the abdomen for the day and then is drained at night.

Insertion of the permanent abdominal catheter is done by the physician in the hospital either in the operating room or at the bedside under local anesthesia. Apparatus for CAPD includes the dialysis solution, as determined by physician according to the patient's need, as well as transfer sets connecting the dialysate to the dialysis catheter and connectors to make the connections with the transfer sets and the dialysate solution. Apparatus for CCPD includes the cycler machine, dialysis solution, and the CCPD connections. Complications of peritoneal dialysis include catheter problems such as displacement, leakage and plugging, bowel or bladder perforation, peritonitis, catheter tunnel infections, and pain.

The primary **caretaker** needs to be able to take the child to the hospital/clinic for periodic examinations and blood drawing. The caretaker needs to be trained in the care of the catheter; the assembly of the apparatus and the dialysate with aseptic technique; and the signs and symptoms of peritonitis or other complications. For further information about dialysis, see: Daugirdas and Ing (1988); Friedman (1984); LePontois, Moel, and Cohn (1987); and Binkley (1984).

ENDOCRINOLOGICAL PROBLEMS

The most common endocrinological disorder requiring home care is Diabetes Mellitus affecting one in 15 Americans and approximately one in 500 children.

Diabetes Mellitus

Type 1 Diabetes Mellitus (DM) is an inherited disease of a deficiency or complete lack of the hormone, insulin. Insulin, which is made in the pancreas, regulates the movement of glucose (sugar) into the cells. Glucose is the primary fuel used by the body. If the cells do not have glucose, then fat is broken down as the source of energy which will be reflected as ketones in the urine. Diabetics are unable to regulate sugar or fat metabolism without receiving exogenous insulin by injection. Elevated blood glucose and ketones in the urine are two indicators of diabetic ketoacidosis. Diabetic ketoacidosis is the main cause of death and severe illness from this disease. This metabolic derangement can cause nausea, vomiting, dehydration, salt depletion, coma or even death if not treated promptly. Major long term complications of diabetes mellitus are thought to be prevented if not delayed by optimal glucose control. These complications include diabetic retinopathy (eye disease) possibly resulting in blindness; kidney problems possibly causing kidney failure; and nerve problems causing tingling, pain or loss of sensation.

The regulation of glucose in the blood stream within a normal range, by manipulating the amount of exogenous insulin, diet control and exercise is paramount to controlling this disease. There are now portable systems for self or caretaker monitoring of blood glucose that can be used in the home. Blood from a finger prick is placed on the meter. The meter operates by shining a light through the blood, assessing a color change on a strip or measuring a chemical reaction, giving a readout of blood glucose expressed as milligrams per deciliter. Size, time for test result, cost, ease of use, audio readout, calibration, and memory are features which vary with the type of meters. Also available for home use are numerous finger sticking devices used for finger pricks, which are simple, quick, easy to use and cause as little pain as possible. Insulin itself is extracted from many different sources, but human insulin is the one of choice with the strength of insulin being 100 units to one milliliter. Insulins have different onset of action times varying from ½ to six hours, 2–24 hours, and 4–36 hours. Insulin must be injected by a syringe with a small needle into the subcutaneous area under the skin. The usual sites for injection include the thighs, upper arms, hips and abdominal area. Sites of injection are rotated to prevent fat decay under the skin. Some children and caretakers are bothered by giving injections. There are injection aids such as insertion aids, infusers, insulin pens or jet injectors to help in this process. Daily injections is the current means to ensure tight control of glucose. Most children are on a twice a day split mixed (mixture of two different onset of action insulins) dose schedule.

Occasionally, a child will have a reaction to the insulin and the glucose will drop precipitously. Symptoms of hypoglycemia (low blood sugar) include confusion, shakiness, headache, dizziness, sudden hunger or sleepiness. Treatment includes giving the child sugar, fruit juice or regular soft drink. Glucagon, a blood sugar raising hormone, should be given to a child who is unconscious or unable to swallow. This hormone also must be injected.

Urine must be tested to detect the presence of ketones, in the face of an elevated blood sugar and glucose. There are several urine testing products which work by dipping a chemically treated stick into urine, or by placing a drop of urine on a tablet and then reading a color change.

Normal growth and development of children with diabetes mellitus is related to good metabolic control of the disease which primarily means control of glucose metabolism. In addition to insulin, diet can help in this control. With a few exceptions, nutrition requirements for these children are essentially the same as for any child. Calories should be comprised of approximately 55% carbohydrates, 30% fat, and 15% protein. The carbohydrates should be predominantly complex carbohydrates (70%) such as starch and the intake of (simple) sugars should be restricted. The daily diet is constructed to maintain the same amount of calories with the same ratio of food types. The child and caretaker learn how to manipulate the diet so as to maintain a normal blood glucose and at the same time be able to eat the same food the family is eating or what the child likes. Individualization of the diet to the child's food likes and dislikes is strongly associated with compliance to the regimen.

Exercise is helpful in controlling overeating, obesity, and diabetes. In general, people who exercise are healthier and live longer, so exercise should be encouraged. There are no restrictions on exercise for the child with diabetes. The child should be encouraged to participate in school sports programs and other activities.

The **caretaker** must be trained in the signs and symptoms of diabetic ketoacidosis; signs and symptoms of hypoglycemia; diet adjustment; types, schedule and mode of administration of insulin; how to measure blood glucose; how to test for ketones in the urine and then how to change the insulin dose based on the blood sugar; and when to call the physician. Equipment needed includes a meter for self-monitoring of blood glucose and supplies, finger sticking equipment and supplies, urine testing supplies, insulin, glucagon, syringes, alcohol wipes, and other equipment as recommended by the physician. For a further description of diabetes mellitus and diabetes products, see: Tomky, Feder, Betschart, Siminerio, Narins, Weinrauch, Guthrie, Hinnen, Campbell and Stenger (1989); Sperling (1987); and Daniels (1988).

CANCER

The medical care of the child at home with cancer encompasses a wide range of therapies including cancer treatment modalities, nutritional support, oxygen therapy, physical therapy, pain management, day-to-day total body function care, transfusions, antibiotic treatments and psychological support. The family must be both technically and emotionally capable of providing such care before a child goes home from the hospital.

Cancer chemotherapy may include giving medication by mouth, by injection into the subcutaneous space or via a central line. Nutritional support may be delivered by N/G, G-tube or TPN as described earlier. For a child in pain, the caretaker may be required to give pain medicine orally or as injection into the muscle or through a central line in a continuous or periodic mode. Types, range of amount and schedules of medications are predetermined by the physician. Occasionally, timing and amount of pain relieving medication are left to the discretion of the child and caretaker. Antibiotic treatment, blood, and platelet transfusions can occur in the home by way of the central line.

Caretakers may need to be trained in the proper care of the nutritional line and/or the central line catheter, administration of medications, and signs and symptoms of infection. Depending on the condition of the child, the caretakers may need to perform basic nursing care in the home such as giving bed baths, oral hygiene care, skin care, changing an occupied bed, transferring the patient from bed to chair, use of a bed pan or urinal, dealing with nausea and loss of appetite.

The stress of having a child with cancer may produce in families guilt, fear, anger, frustration, and denial in family members; which may lead to depression and poor coping skills. Further, interpersonal relationships with family members may become dysfunctional. Hospital and community support systems are essential and should be in place once the initial diagnosis is made in the hospital and continued when the child goes home.

If the child is terminally ill, issues of death and dying must be addressed. The goal of care should be to minimize the suffering of the patient and their families. Parents may want their child to die with dignity and peace at home rather than in the hospital. Studies have shown that parents and siblings of patients receiving a comprehensive home care program adjusted better to the death of the child than families whose child died in the hospital. Every effort should be made to respect and comply with the wishes of the child and his/her family. For further description of cancer and death and dying issues, see: Mulhern, Lauer, and Hoffmann (1983); Edstrom & Miller (1981); Michielutte, Patterson and Herndon (1981); Monaco (1986); Bubela (1981); and Freund and Siegel (1986).

HEMATOLOGY

The most common hematological disease requiring home treatment is sickle cell disease. The disease effects nearly one in five hundred Black Americans.

Sickle Cell Disease

Sickle Cell Disease is an inherited chronic anemia affecting the hemoglobin in the red blood cells. Hemoglobin is the molecule in red blood cells that carries oxygen from the lung to the cells in all parts of the body. Under certain conditions, when the abnormal hemoglobin gives up the oxygen, the cells will become sickled in shape instead of remaining in the typical donut configuration. The two factors which cause the problems in children with sickle cell disease include the sickled red blood cells and the anemia. The sickled cells can jam or block blood in the blood vessels resulting in 1) painful bone crises predominantly in the hands, feet, long bones, and soft tissue, 2) acute abdominal pain, 3) pulmonary infarcts (an area in the lung that has died because of inadequate blood supply), 4) cerebral vascular accidents, and 5) priapism (persistent erection of the penis caused by blockage of blood by the sickled cells). Other complications of this disease include 1) splenic cell sequestration where the sickled cells block the blood from the spleen causing the spleen to trap large amounts of blood in it; 2) aplastic crisis caused by a viral or bacterial infection producing a temporary cessation of bone marrow activity where production of the white and red blood cells occurs, and 3) infections. Infections are the most common cause of death in children with sickle cell anemia. Certain bacterial infections are more frequent and severe in children with sickle cell disease. The reason for the increased susceptibility are defects in the child's immunity system. Anemia is caused by the body's removal of the abnormal sickled cells resulting in a decreased number of cells to carry hemoglobin. Signs and symptoms of anemia are lack of energy, poor appetite, and slower growth.

Babies who inherit one abnormal gene from a parent which produces the sickle hemoglobin, will have sickle cell trait. Babies who inherit two abnormal genes, one from each parent, will have sickle cell anemia, the disease. Sickle cell trait occurs in one in 12 black Americans. Children with sickle cell trait are healthy and rarely have any problems. The knowledge that one has sickle cell trait is important when the adult with sickle cell trait is thinking about having his/her own child and passing on the abnormal gene. Signs and symptoms of sickle cell anemia usually do not appear until after six months of age. A newborn's blood is screened shortly after birth to assess if the child has the disease. If the child has the disease, he/she is put on penicillin prophylactically to prevent overwhelming bacterial infections.

The two most common acute problems which need to be medically managed are infections and painful bony crises. A child with a temperature greater than 38.5 degrees Centigrade (100.5 degrees Fahrenheit) must be seen by a physician promptly. The child will be assessed by the physician for possible infection and either be sent home on antibiotics or admitted to the hospital. A painful bony crisis can be started by infection, fatigue, unusual stress, over exertion, high altitudes or other factors. These vaso-occlusive crises must be treated with potent drugs to relieve the pain, bed rest, and increased fluid intake. This management is started in the home. If the pain is not relieved or tolerated, the child may come to the hospital for stronger pain relieving medications. Some children may need to be admitted to the hospital for these medications. Sickle Cell Disease is quite variable among children; some may have few and only mild problems while others may have frequent and severe complications.

Caretakers need to be trained to recognize the signs and symptoms of all the complications that can arise from this disease. They should be taught how to feel for a spleen in young children. They need to give the children daily prophylactic antibiotics. They need to be taught how to respond to fever or other signs or symptoms of infections. Caretakers need to make sure that children drink plenty of fluids, especially in the summer, dress warmly in the winter, and prevent over exertion in play. They must have prompt and frequent access to health care professionals that treat children with Sickle Cell Disease. Further they must be trained to administer potent pain relieving medications. For further description of Sickle Cell Disease, see: Pearson (1987); Platt and Nathan (1987); National Association for Sickle Cell Disease (1974); and Fosnot (1978).

INFECTIOUS DISEASES

Infectious diseases requiring intravenous (IV) or intramuscular (IM) administration of antibiotics have generally been treated in the hospital. However, there is a trend to complete antibiotic treatment in the home after the infection has been controlled in the hospital. This trend has come about due to the advances in antibiotic therapy and the availability of visiting nurse service, home therapy teams, and parental education in administering antibiotics. For home therapy to be effective, the child must continue to have close follow up with the physician and that the child receive antibiotics in the home. The two main infectious diseases that have been treated at home include osteomyelitis and septic arthritis.

Osteomyelitis

Osteomyelitis is a bacterial infection of the bone usually requiring up to six to eight weeks of antibiotic therapy. The initial mode of administration of the antibiotic is usually IV (or occasionally IM). After improvement in both the clinical signs and laboratory values such as the sedimentation rate, the patient may be sent home to continue on antibiotic treatment by IV, IM, or oral route. If there is extensive bone destruction or concern about a pathologic fracture, the bone may be immobilized in a cast. If immobilization is necessary, exercise of the joints out of the cast daily may be needed to prevent contractures. Thus, physical therapy may be needed. A small proportion of patients will develop chronic osteomyelitis because the infection was not diagnosed or treated early, or was not completely eradicated by antibiotics. Non-compliance may also result in chronic osteomyelitis. If chronic osteomyelitis occurs, antibiotics may be required for months, and surgical debridement may be needed as well.

Septic Arthritis

Septic arthritis is a bacterial infection of a joint. Treatment is similar to that for osteomyelitis, although surgical drainage of the joint, especially the hip, is more often necessary to prevent damage to cartilage, the covering of the end of bones. As the clinical condition improves, completion of the six to eight week course of antibiotics can be given in the home, together with physical therapy to regain mobility.

Caretakers require training in administering IV, IM or oral antibiotics; the importance of compliance; how to recognize signs and symptoms of increasing infection; and how to exercise the joints. Equipment needs include IV pole, intravenous needles, and IV starting equipment. For further description of antibiotic therapy in the home see: May (1984); Harris, Buckle and Coffey (1986).

Meningitis

Meningitis is an inflammation of the meninges which are the three membranes which line the brain and the spinal cord. The inflammation can be caused by several infectious agents including bacteria or viruses. Bacterial meningitis is a serious infection and prompt treatment with antibiotic therapy in the hospital is important to prevent death and brain damage. Once the child improves clinically, some physicians choose to complete the antibiotic therapy at home. The decision to treat the child in the home is based on the child's clinical condition, the reliability of the parents to assess the child's medical condition and to follow instructions, and the availability of the visiting nurse service or home therapy team to assess the patient and administer antibiotics if necessary.

Caretakers require training in administering IV, IM, or oral antibiotics; the importance of compliance; and how to recognize signs and symptoms of increasing infection. Equipment needed includes IV pole, IV needles, and IV starting equipment. For further description of treatment of meningitis at home, see: Giebink, Hall, Lepow and Plotkin (1988).

Contagious Diseases

The following two contagious diseases may have major impact on the transition of children to home care. These diseases pose a risk of infecting family members with a potential life threatening illness. These two infectious viral agents are Hepatitis B Virus (HBV) and Human Immunodeficiency Virus (HIV). There is no way to eradicate either virus.

Hepatitis

Hepatitis is an inflammation of the liver caused by several agents including HBV. The severity and duration of Hepatitis B, which is caused by HBV, is variable. Usually, the disease is a mild, self-limited illness with nonspecific symptoms. However, approximately 1% of those infected with Hepatitis B viral infection develop fulminant hepatitis and die. Ten per cent of those who recover from an acute hepatitis infection become chronic carriers of the virus. The chronic carriers do not have an active infection but continue to shed the virus in their blood, feces and secretions and pose a source of contagion to the family. Mothers who have the HBV can transmit the virus to their newborn babies at delivery. These babies may develop hepatitis and may become chronic carriers of the virus. Home health issues concern the contagion problem.

To prevent spread of this virus, precautions for handling blood and body fluids should be instituted, especially hand washing after contact with the child and the wearing of disposable rubber gloves for touching blood or body fluids. Hepatitis B has a low level of communicability from saliva, urine, or feces. Commercially available cleaners are used for cleaning of spills of bodily secretions or blood on surfaces. Disposable towels or tissues should be used when possible. Family members and other persons considered to be at high risk for exposure to the virus should receive Hepatitis B vaccines. A series of two or three injections are given over a specific delineated time frame. There are very few side effects of the vaccine and it confers protection for at least five years. With appropriate precautions and receiving of the Hepatitis B vaccine, family members should be protected from getting Hepatitis B virus.

Caretakers require training in methods of controlling the contagion. All family members should receive Hepatitis B vaccine with boosters every five years. Equipment needed includes disposable rubber gloves, disposable towels, and commercial cleaning liquid.

Acquired Immunodeficiency Syndrome (AIDS)

Acquired Immunodeficiency Syndrome (AIDS) is caused by the HIV. HIV infection gradually and progressively affects the human host

defense mechanism and renders the patient defenseless and suscep-
tible to opportunistic infections and malignancies. The spectrum of
HIV infection ranges broadly from asymptomatic, to enlarged lymph
nodes with immunocompromise without infection, to symptomatic
disease with infection. Most infected children are likely to have acquired this infection through birth from HIV-positive mothers or
through contaminated blood or blood products.

Diagnosis of this infection is based on clinical and laboratory findings. One of the laboratory tests measures antibodies to this virus in
the blood. Mothers with HIV-antibodies may passively transfer their
antibodies to the newborn infant. In the majority of these infants,
the antibodies measured in the infant from birth to 15 months of age
may be the mother's antibodies. These children have no symptoms.
However, if the antibodies persist after 15 months of age and/or signs
or symptoms of this disease occur during this age period, the child is
likely to be infected with the virus and may develop the full spectrum
of AIDS.

Home health care issues revolve around contagion, medical care,
and death and dying issues. There have been no reports of transmission from a HIV-infected child to other individuals in the household setting, nor transmission in day care settings or acquisition of
the virus by foster parents. Reported transmission has been solely by
sexual contact or by blood transmission. As with Hepatitis B virus,
the same precautions for handling of blood and body secretions are
needed. Family and community education is often needed to prevent
social isolation. Ungloved touching and cuddling is safe and encouraged. There is no cure for AIDS. Medical treatment of children with
AIDS consists in treating resulting opportunistic infections and secondary malignancies. Psychosocial support for the family and child
about death and dying is essential.

Caretakers require training to administer intravenous, intramuscular, or oral antibiotics or medicines; how to control for contagion;
how to deal with community issues; and how to advocate for the
child. Caretakers need psychosocial support for themselves and for
the child during times of stress, crisis, and around death and dying
issues. Respite care is often essential. Equipment needed includes
intravenous apparatus with IV starting paraphernalia, disposable rubber gloves and paper towels, and commercial cleaning liquid. For
further description of infectious diseases, see: Peter, Hall, Lepow
and Phillips (1988); Harris, Buckle and Coffey (1986); and American
Academy of Pediatrics, Task Force on Pediatrics AIDS (1989).

ORTHOPEDIC PROBLEMS

Home care for orthopedic problems usually consist of care of child with limb cast, full body cast (spica) or traction. Limb cast care involves keeping the cast clean and dry and assessing the limb for color, temperature, swelling and pain. Children can be in limb casts anywhere from a few weeks to up to 12 weeks. Children in spica casts are usually positioned in prone for feeding, muscle stretching, and developmental purposes. Children are usually in spica casts for 3, 6, or as long as 12 weeks.

Traction at home has been shown to be as effective as hospital traction in the management of congenital dislocation of the hip. Medical care involves the placement of longitudinal skin traction of the lower extremity with weight application of two to ten pounds depending on the child's age and tolerance. Usual duration of traction is approximately six weeks.

The **caretaker** must learn how to apply the traction correctly, and be knowledgeable in the prevention of skin breakdown at the site of application and of decubitus ulcers. Equipment needs include the traction apparatus and a bed with a foot board. For further description of home traction, see: Voutsinas, MacEwen and Boos (1984).

CARDIAC PROBLEMS

Among children, the most common heart problems are congenital. Born with structural abnormalities of the heart, many children will require surgical intervention to ameliorate or correct their lesions. Home therapy may include emphasis on nutrition with special formulas or alternative modes of feeding (as discussed earlier). If the infant is cyanotic (blue), the child may need oxygen, usually delivered by nasal cannula. Most of these children will be on medications including a diuretic, digoxin and prophylactic antibiotics for dental interventions.

Children with acquired heart problems, usually caused by infections, may require long term antibiotics. Other modalities of treatment needed may include cardiac medications, bed rest, and prophylactic antibiotics for dental interventions.

Children with arrhythmias (irregular heart rate) may be on cardiac medications or need a cardiac pacer to control the arrhythmias. Caretakers may need periodically to monitor the child's heart rate by using a stethescope to count the heart beats. These children can also be transtelephonically monitored by the heart station at a medical center.

For children with heart problems, **caretakers** need to be trained in nutritional care, medication schedules, oxygen delivery, the use of the stethescope, the signs and symptoms of cardiac failure, and what to do in case of emergency. For further information concerning children's heart disease, see: Moller, Neal and Hoffman (1987).

CONCLUSION

At present, there appears to be no limit to the growth of technology. In the future, hospitals will be occupied only by the very sickest of children and homes will become once again the traditional site for health care. Financial and humane pressure to care for stable but medically complex children in the home will increase. At the same time, however, the supply of medically trained professionals is not expected to keep up with the increasing demand. Therefore, parents and alternative caretakers will be required to account for more and more of the hands-on health care formerly provided by nurses, respiratory therapists, occupational therapists, physical therapists, and speech therapists. By the twenty-first century, we will have come full circle back to the model, but not to the methods, of the family-centered home health care that has characterized most of human history.

REFERENCES

Alltop, S. A. (1988). Teaching for discharge: Gastrostomy tubes. *RN*, 42–46.

American Academy of Pediatrics, Ad Hoc Task Forces on Home Care of Chronically Ill Infants and Children. (1984). Guidelines for home care of infants, children, and adolescents with chronic disease. *Pediatrics, 74* (3), 434–436.

American Academy of Pediatrics, Committee on Children with Disabilities. (1986). Transition of severely disabled children from hospital or chronic care facilities to the community. *Pediatrics, 78* (3), 531–534.

American Academy of Pediatrics, Committee on Infectious Diseases. (1988). Treatment of bacterial meningitis. *Pediatrics, 81* (6), 904–907.

American Academy of Pediatrics, Task Force on Pediatrics AIDS. (1989). Infants and children with acquired immuno-deficiency syndrome: Placement in adoption and foster care. *Pediatrics, 83* (4), 609–612.

Ariagno, R. L. (1984). Evaluation and management of infantile apnea. *Pediatric Annals, 13* (3), 210–217.

Ariagno, R. L. & Glotzbach, S. F. (1987). Home monitoring of high-risk infants. *Chest, 91* (6), 898–900.

Association for the Care of Children's Health. (1984). *Home care for children with serious handicapping conditions.* (A Report on a Conference Sponsored by the Association for the Care of Children's Health and the Division of Maternal and Child Health, Public Health Service, U.S. Department of Health and Human Services, Houston, TX). Washington, D.C.: Author.

Association for the Care of Children's Health. (1988). *From hospital to home care: An annotated bibliography.* Washington, D.C.: Author.

Barber, J. R. (1984). Home parenteral nutrition. *Minnesota Pharmacist,* 6–11.

Batshaw, M. L. & Perret, Y. M. (1987). *Children with handicaps: A medical primer.* Baltimore: Paul H. Brookes Publishing Co.

Binkley, L. S. (1984). Keeping up with peritoneal dialysis. *American Journal of Nursing,* 729–733.

Bleck, E. E. & Nagel, D. A. (Eds.). (1982). *Physically handicapped children, American atlas for teachers,* New York: Grune and Stratton, Inc.

Brown, L. W. (1984) Home monitoring of the high-risk infant. *Clinics in Perinatology, 11* (1), 85–99.

Bubela, N. (1981). Technical and psychological problems and concerns arising from the outpatient treatment of cancer with direct intraarterial infusion. *Cancer Nursing,* 305–309.

Burr, B. H., Guyer, B., Todres, I. D., Abrahams, B., & Chiodo, T. (1983). Home care for children on respirators. *New England Journal of Medicine, 309* (21), 1319–1323.

Cunningham, J. C. & Taussig, L. M. (1989). *A guide to cystic fibrosis for parents and children.* Bethesda, Maryland: Cystic Fibrosis Foundation.

Daniels, D. R. (1988). A guide to pediatric diabetes for the home health nurse. *Home Health Care Nurse, 6* (5), 22–26.

Daugirdas, J. T. & Ing, T. S. (Eds.). (1988). *Handbook of dialysis.* Boston: Little, Brown and Co.

Donati, M. A., Guenette, G., & Auerbach, H. (1987). Prospective controlled study of home and hospital therapy of cystic fibrosis pulmonary disease. *Journal of Pediatrics, 111* (1), 28–33.

Edstrom, S., & Miller, M. W. (1981). Preparing the family to care for the cancer patient: A home care course. *Cancer Nursing,* 49–52.

Fischer, D. A. (1985). Long-term management of the ventilator patient in the home. *Cleveland Clinic Quarterly, 52* (3), 303–306.

Fosnot, H. (Ed.). (1978). *Sickle cell disease. Tell the facts-quell the fables.* National Association for Sickle Cell Disease, Inc., Darien, CT: Patient Care Publications.

Foster, S., & Hoskins, D. (1981). Home care of the child with a tracheotomy tube. *Pediatric Clinics of North America, 28* (4), 855–857.

Freund, B. L. & Siegel, K. (1986). Problems in transition following bone marrow transplantation: Psychosocial aspects. *American Journal of Orthopsychiatry, 56* (2), 244–252.

Friedman, E. A. (1984). Critical appraisal of continuous ambulatory peritoneal dialysis. *Annual Review of Medicine, 35*, 233–248.

Garber, H. P. & Balas-Stevens, S. (1984). A discharge tool for teaching parents to monitor infant apnea at home, *Maternal and Child Nursing, 9*, 178–180.

Goldenhersh, M. J. & Rachelefsky, G. S. (1989). Childhood asthma: Overview. *Pediatrics in Review, 10* (8), 227–234.

Gullate, M. M. (1989). Managing an implanted infusion device. *RN*, 45–49.

Halpern, R. (1986). Home-based early intervention: Dimensions of current practice. *Child Welfare, 65* (4), 387–398.

Hanson, J. (Ed.). (1987). *Parent guide to bronchopulmonary dysplasia (BPD).* New Mexico: American Lung Association.

Harper, T. B. & Strunk, R. C. (1981). Techniques of administration of metered-dose aerosolized drugs in asthmatic children. *American Journal of Diseases of Children, 135*, 218–221.

Harris, L. F., Buckle, T. F., & Coffey, F. L. (1986). Intravenous Antibiotics at Home. *Southern Medical Journal, 79* (2), 193–196.

Hazinski, M. F. (1986). Pediatric home tracheostomy care: A parent's guide. *Pediatric Nursing, 12* (1), 41–69.

LePontois, J., Moel, D. I., & Cohn, R. A. (1987). Family adjustment to pediatric ambulatory dialysis. *American Journal of Orthopsychiatry, 57* (1), 78–83.

Lucas, J., Golish, J., Sleeper, G., & O'Ryan, J. A. (Eds.). (1988). *Home respiratory care.* Norwalk: Appleton & Lange.

Mapp, C. S. (1988). Trach care: Are you aware of all the dangers? *Nursing, 18* (7), 34–42.

May, C. (1984). Antibiotic therapy at home. *American Journal of Nursing*, 348–349.

McBride, J. T. (1984). Infantile apnea. *Pediatrics in Review, 5* (9), 275–284.

Michielutte, R., Patterson, R. B., and Herndon, A. (1981). Evaluation of a home visitation program for families of children with cancer. *American Journal of Pediatric Hematology/Oncology, 3* (3), 239–245.

Moller, J. H., Neal, W. A., & Hoffman, W. R. (1987). *A parent's guide to heart disorders*. Minneapolis: University of Minnesota Press.

Monaco, G. P. (1986). Resources available to the family of the child with cancer. *Cancer, 58*, (2), 516–521.

Mulhern, R. K., Lauer, M. E., & Hoffmann, R. G. (1983). Death of a child at home or in the hospital: Subsequent psychological adjustment of the family. *Pediatrics, 71* (5), 743–747.

National Association for Sickle Cell Disease, Inc. (1974). *How to help your child to "take it in stride": Advice for parents of children with sickle cell anemia*. Los Angeles, CA.

Norris-Berkemeyer, S. & Hutchins, K. H. (1986). Home apnea monitoring. *Pediatric Nursing, 12* (4), 259–304.

O'Donohue, W. J., Giovannoni, R. M., Keens, T. G., & Plummer, A. L. (1986). Long-term mechanical ventilation: Guidelines for management in the home and at alternate community sites. *Chest, 90* (1): 1S–37S.

O'Ryan, J. A. & Burns, D. G. (1984). *Pulmonary rehabilitation: From hospital to home*. Chicago: Year Book Medical Publishers, Inc.

Okamoto, E., Fee, W. E., Boles, R., Calcaterra, T. C., Dobie, R. A., & Steadman, M. G. (1977). Safety of hospital vs. home care of infant tracheotomies. *Tr American Academy of Ophthalmology and Otolaryngology, 84*, 92–99.

Paarlberg, J. & Balint, J. P. (1985). Gastrostomy tubes: Practical guidelines for home care. *Pediatric Nursing*, 99–102.

Pearson, H. A. (1987). Sickle Cell Diseases: Diagnosis and Management in Infancy and Childhood. *Pediatics in Review 9* (4), 121–130.

Perry, M. A. and Hayes, N. M. (1988). Bronchopulmonary dysplasia: Discharge planning and complex home care. *Neonatal Network, 7* (3), 13–17.

Peter, G., Hall, G. B., Lepow, M. & Phillips, C. F. (Eds.). (1988). *Report on the committee on infectious disease* (21st Edition). Elk Grove, IL: American Academy of Pediatrics.

Platt, O. S. & Nathan, D. G. (1987). Sickle Cell Disease. In D. G. Nathan and F. A. Oski (Eds.), *Hematology of Infancy and Childhood* (pp. 655–698). Philadelphia: W. B. Saunders Co.

Rachelefsky, G. S. (1984). The wheezing child. *Pediatric Patient Education*, 941–947.

Rivard, W. A. (1989). *Home parenteral nutrition instruction manual for parents*. (Available from [Pediatric Nutrition Support Service, Wyler Children's Hospital, University of Chicago Medical Center, 5841 Maryland Avenue, Chicago, IL 60637]).

Russman, B. S. (1983). Early intervention for the biologically handicapped infant and young child: Is it of value? *Pediatrics in Review*, 5 (2), 51–55.

Schreiner, M. S., Donar, M. E., & Kettrick, R. G. (1987). Pediatric home mechanical ventilation. *Pediatric Clinics of North America*, 34 (1), 47–60.

Sperling, M. A. (1987). Outpatient management of diabetes mellitus. *Pediatric Clinics of North America*, 34 (4), 919–934.

Stein, R. E. K. & Jessop, D. J. (1984). Does pediatric home care make a difference for children with chronic illness? Findings from the pediatric ambulatory care treatment study. *Pediatrics*, 73 (6), 845–853.

Stern, R. C. (1989). The primary care physician and the patient with cystic fibrosis. *Journal of Pediatrics*, 114 (1), 31–36.

Taft, L. T. (1984). Cerebral palsy. *Pediatrics in Review*, 6 (2), 35–45.

Tomky, D., Feder, A. S., Betschart, J., Siminerio, L., Narins, B., Weinrauch, S., Guthrie, D. W., Hinnen, D., Campbell, K., & Stenger, P. D. (1989). 1990 buyer's guide to diabetes products. *Diabetes Forecast*, 42 (10), 43–82.

Voutsinas, S. A., MacEwen, G. D., & Boos, M. L. (1984). Home traction in the management of congenital dislocation of the hip. *Archives of Orthopedic Trauma Surgery*, 102, 135–140.

Wasserman, A. L. (1984). A prospective study of the impact of home monitoring on the family. *Pediatrics*, 74 (3), 323–329.

Wheeler, W. B. & Colten, H. R. (1988). Cystic fibrosis: Current approach to diagnosis and management. *Pediatrics in Review*, 9 (8), 241–248.

CHAPTER 4

FROM INTENSIVE CARE UNIT TO HOME: THE ROLE OF PEDIATRIC TRANSITIONAL CARE

MARK J. MERKENS

INTRODUCTION

A Changing Patient Population

The face of hospital-based pediatrics of the early 1990's has changed. Medical professionals and non-medical persons alike would be struck upon visiting a regional pediatric medical center by the apparent change in the complexion and spectrum of diseases and treatments. Intensive care and surgery for the pediatric-age patient has come of age. Technology marches on: a visit to the pediatric ward reveals children treated with hyperalimentation, ventilation, antiviral respiratory therapies, immune therapy and organ transplant. In short, new treatments and procedures allow the rescue of children who could not have been saved as recently as a decade ago.

Simultaneously the spectrum of diagnoses recorded in the medical records of children treated in today's tertiary pediatric wards has changed. Certain catastrophic entities have waned, to be replaced by others. Gone is Reye's Syndrome, replaced by children surviving complex congenital conditions, horrendous accidents, AIDS and other severe chronic illnesses.

Yet old problems have new meanings. Basic science research has yielded improvements in care of chronic illnesses, prolonging life expectancy. Whereas the mean survival with cystic fibrosis in 1970 was 7 years, a child with the same diagnosis could have expected to live to seventeen in 1980, and now would have half a chance to live into their twenties. The prevalence rate of most chronic illnesses now equals the incidence: most children with chronic illness now survive into adulthood.

To round out the current complexion, British demographers describe our population as in the midst of a second or "mini-bulge."
Children of the post-war baby boom are bearing children.

Our visit to a hypothetical pediatric ward has clarified that more
children are living longer with both familiar and new medical problems. And the state of health of many of these children can be understood as changed by current therapies. Most children treated with
intensive care die or recover. Some, however, don't—they are rescued, but cannot be restored to perfect health. Mere survival may
be dependent upon the continued function of a mechanical or phar-
macological intervention. Such a condition may be perceived as a
new state of health—stable, but dependent upon current technology
for life. For the rest of that child's life. Such children must be viewed
as stable, but dependent upon current high level technology for survival. Biologic stability may be labile, or dependent upon the continued function of equipment or receipt of therapies. Current vogue
is to label such children as medically fragile or technology-dependent.
The U.S. Congressional Office of Technology Assessment (1987)
projects on a national level as many as 100,000 children who are
technology dependent.

These cases present ethical problems unlike those of elderly who
may be receiving the same therapies. Typically the child's condition
is not terminal. The long-term prognosis perhaps cannot be projected.
Many have normal mental capacities. It would be unethical, if not
immoral, to remove the specific therapy or technology that continues
to support life itself.

The severity of the acute condition, the duration of successful recuperation, and prolonged technology-dependency may have neces-
sitated weeks of hospitalization. The number of severely chronically
ill and handicapped children who are hospitalized more than ninety
days in tertiary care hospitals is growing. These children require
twenty-four hour nursing care including monitoring and observation.

The irony of the Gordian knot these cases present is that many of
the therapies required were designed to be provided only in an intensive care unit. After months of instability and efforts to wean from
the technological support, the child may become stable but indefinitely dependent upon the extra technology. Such cases occupy beds
in intensive care units where costs are in excess of $1,000 per day.
These patients may make up only 7% of all children admitted to the
Pediatric Intensive Care Unit (P.I.C.U.), but consume approximately
50% of all P.I.C.U. resources (Pollack, Wilkinson, & Glass, 1987).

The Impact of Prolonged Hospitalization

Hospitals are designed for efficient delivery of medical care, not as environments for children to grow in. Imagine the impact of prolonged hospitalization upon a child's development. Because saving lives goes on around the clock, an intensive care unit has no diurnal patterns. Noise levels as well as stress are high. A child-patient receives aberrant social stimulation and little opportunity for age-appropriate play and motor activities. Normal social interaction, bonding and parenting are eschewed. In the unhealthy social environment of the I.C.U. a child learns erroneous interaction with adult medical staff during stressful situations such as medical emergencies in adjacent patients. Staff may become emotionally bonded to their patient. Having literally saved the child's life, medical and nursing personnel may prejudicially perceive themselves as better qualified in child rearing than the biologic parents. Parents who must commute to be with their hospitalized child find their home life suffering. In short, hospitals are pathological environments for children to be in.

A PROPOSED SOLUTION: TRANSITIONAL CARE

Perceptive medical staff or demanding parents will seek to have a child's care transferred out of the intensive care unit and eventually to home or the best alternative residential environment. Success will require revised perception of the patient's condition, redirection of staff philosophy toward enablement, and discharge planning.

Despite the required use of oxygen, therapies, medications, equipment, or electronic monitors, the child's condition may be unchanging for long periods. Efforts to wean the child's body from these dependencies may be futile or contraindicated in the short term. But because infants continue to grow such tissues as lung alveoli and brain cells, the potential for eventual independence may be real. The course of a previously unknown condition must be viewed as potentially improving.

Transitional care is directed at this population of children. *Pediatric transitional care is a program providing a broad range of medical and non-medical services needed to promote the optimal development of children with severe chronic illnesses and handicapping conditions, especially those who are medically fragile or dependent upon high technology interventions* (Merkens, 1983). Pediatric transitional care is particularly directed at children who reside long-term in acute care hospitals—children perhaps receiving a higher level of medical and nursing care than they require at unnecessarily high cost, and who may have experienced detrimental effects from long-term hospitalization. These children need a host of non-medical services and developmentally oriented environment often not provided in either intensive hospital or custodial care settings. Pediatric transitional care is best understood as a "level between": acute care hospitalization and home, or acute care hospitalization and custodial care. Pediatric transitional care is focused on support of the child's developmental needs and those of the family which have been stressed with significant emotional and financial pressures.

Hospital rules and regulations may require that certain medical interventions be provided only in an intensive care unit. But such requirements may be based only on their use in unstable medical conditions. As the child's condition remains unchanging for long periods, otherwise extreme medical interventions may be safely used in less intensive environments. For example, anesthesia rules may prohibit patients on ventilators to be housed anywhere but in an I.C.U. The child whose medical condition has not changed for over a month must be perceived as stable, despite high level technology dependency. Dependency is not equivalent to severity or acuteness. The child who is respiratory dependent may be stable enough to be moved to a stepdown unit, regular ward, and eventually to home and the community. Regulations will need revision to allow such new approaches.

The overall goal of transitional care is normalization of the child and his family in as many aspects of life as possible. The objective is to alter all the negative outcomes of hospitalization which we have highlighted. The means to reach that end include revising usual hospital practice of care provision, provision of developmentally appropriate activities, and family support. The underlying philosophy is that the parents and family own the child, not the medical center and staff. The child is to be moved to the "least restrictive environment"for care and growth, and assumption of care by the family or its surrogate. In other words, the ultimate objective is discharge from hospital to home or the best alternative environment. That must be based upon the child and family strengths and is carried out by increasing assumption of care by parents (foster or biologic), and other community providers.

The products of pediatric transitional care are a series of outcomes new to the acute hospital. One outcome is achievement of the new philosophy fostered by the Surgeon General of the U.S.: *family-centered care* (Brewer, McPherson, Magrab, & Hutchins, 1989). Another is all the steps necessary for discharge from tertiary hospital. Training of local community providers can be expanded beyond the individual child to address the overall issues presented by these children who are technology dependent and medically fragile.

Patients Served

Five groups of children with chronic illness who would benefit from transitional care can be identified (La Rabida, 1984).

The first group the transitional unit serves are those requiring twenty-four hour nursing care as well as treatment, monitoring, observation, and the use of various equipment and technologies for the maintenance of medical stability. These are, therefore, children whose chronic condition makes them medically fragile and technology dependent patients. The number of ventilator-supported children in the Chicago region was the impetus for starting the Chronic Illness Transitional Unit at La Rabida Children's Hospital and Research Center, of the University of Chicago in 1983. Children with bronchopulmonary dysplasia including oxygen dependency and bronchospasm were soon cared for there. Such a unit would also be an excellent setting to care for children needing renal dialysis or hyperalimentation.

A second group of other, less ill children is cared for in a transitional unit. Children with mild or moderately severe chronic illness needing a change in medical management, application of new equipment or procedure for care, or adaptation counseling benefit from temporary residence with specialized programming in a transitional unit. A child with diabetes in need of a new regimen or temporary removal from home and therapeutic counseling would be well served here.

Children recovering from complicated surgery or severe accident or whose illness involves prolonged recuperation would be developmentally stimulated during recuperation by a transitional program rather than stifled by hospitalization.

A fourth group is composed of children "in transition" from tertiary centers to home. Parents and care givers need a setting in which to learn the technical and developmental aspects of their care and management. This process may require weeks, and the unit will be an excellent center for that preparation to take place efficiently.

A fifth group of children who would be specifically targeted to be served by a transitional program: clients of child welfare agencies.

These are children whose basic medical condition is stable and who don't need further hospitalization, but have not been discharged because they wouldn't receive adequate care in their home. An example is a child whose medical condition *could* be maintained by capable parents, residing in an adequate structure, with the availability of necessary services and insurance. However, children under our current consideration are those whose parents are unavailable, inadequate, incapable, unstable, neglectful, abandoning, or abusive. The home structure may be inadequate and unalterable. Finances may be insufficient. Foster care might be indicated for some other reason. Such children are cared for in the transitional unit until the social situation is evaluated and ajudicated, foster parents identified and trained, and home and community services prepared.

There is another generic category of children who may become clients of child welfare agencies even after successful home placement has been arranged or established. Family structure might be altered as a result of illness or death of a parent or adult care taker. The source of income or insurance may be lost. Family coping may collapse under the burden of home care. Okamato and Shurtleff (1981) noted that approximately seventeen percent of their spina bifida patients required foster placement each year—and not necessarily the same patients repeatedly. Like the welfare agencies, medical systems need to be prepared to alter the care program as the social and medical status of the family changes.

THE PEDIATRIC TRANSITIONAL CARE PROGRAM

Our response to these issues has been shaped by experience over the last decade or more at the La Rabida Children's Hospital and Research Center. As a chronic care hospital of the Department of Pediatrics, University of Chicago, Pritzker School of Medicine, La Rabida has progressively changed its mission to conform to the changing patterns of chronic medical illness, developmental disability, and physical handicaps in childhood. Our experience has been reported in numerous settings (Merkens & Anderson, 1983; Perrin, Merkens, & Kohrman, 1983; Merkens, 1984; Merkens, 1990). These discussions are a summary report of those experiences.

We became involved in the plight of the ventilator-dependent child in 1982 following a conference of pediatric department chairman from the Chicago area. The conference was stimulated by the board of

Table 4.1. Objectives of the Pediatric Transitional Care Program.*

A. *Patient care*, including:
    1. Maintenance of medical status.
    2. Maintenance of psychosocial status of child and family.
    3. Habilitation of the child (enablement of the functional abilities of daily living to the best of his/her ability).
    4. Training of home care givers.
    5. Training of community providers.
    6. Followup care of the child and family.
    7. Respite care.
B. *Teaching*
    1. Health care providers in training.
    2. Home care providers.
    3. Community providers.
    4. Continuing education for practicing professionals.
C. *Research*
    1. Demonstration project.
    2. Generic issues faced by these children and their families.
    3. Equipment used for transitional and home care.

*At La Rabida Children's Hospital and Research Center.

directors of a trust, who asked chairmen to address unresolved complex patient care needs. By informal survey it was noted that over twenty intensive care beds were occupied by children who were ventilator-dependent. The trust accepted the recommendation of the chairmen to underwrite the establishment of a model demonstration unit. The trust eventually funded the expanding programs targeted at children with chronic medical illnesses at La Rabida Children's Hospital and Research Center.

During the early part of last decade the problems presented by the ventilator dependent or assisted child was the paradigm of the growing numbers of complex cases highlighted above. It was soon realized that the respiratory dependent child was but one of the children with severe chronic illness who are medically fragile or high technology dependent. Because the considerations directed at this subgroup of children, we will describe the planning process and expand consideration to more generic approaches.

The specific objectives of Pediatric Transitional Care at the La Rabida Children's Hospital are outlined in Table 4.1.

Constructing such a unit is neither possible nor necessary for every tertiary medical center or referral region. But aspects of the comprehensive unit, including equipment, staff, policies and procedures, and above all the program to achieve transition may be adopted according to local resources. Let us consider these aspects separately.

The Transitional Care Unit: The Physical Plant

Transitional care is most effectively provided within a separate ward or even a free-standing facility. Not only is a separate staff inculcated with a philosophy of care, but separate policies and procedures are required. Spread of nosocomial infection into the unit and transfer of abnormal flora from chronic respiratory patients to other patients via staff is restricted. Equipment and layout conducive to the program objectives are built and acquired. The overall concept of transition is thereby literally expressed in concrete.

A total of two hundred square feet surface area per patient must be planned in this unit. One hundred square feet must surround the bed itself, allowing access for staff, equipment, and transport vehicles. The rest of the surface area is composed of usual and customary services such as clean and dirty utility, storage, and staff station. A treatment room is necessary for performance of invasive medical procedures.

The layout will be innovative in a fashion to foster patient privacy and independence. Private and semiprivate rooms are a transition between a sterile open I.C.U. environment to home. The patient will no longer be cared for in a large single room with simple curtains for separation. Instead, patients in transition reside in individual rooms. Crises, medical procedures, and personal conversation can be carried out in confidence. As visual observation and monitoring will be emphasized, there will be much glass area and wide doors allowing staff to see each patient from anywhere within the unit; blinds will be placed so as to allow patient control of privacy. Space and layout will welcome the presence of parents or guardians for bonding as well as training and thereby enhance transfer of care to them.

Construction will similarly foster normalcy. Sound insulation will limit hospital noises and allow for undisturbed sleeping during nap time and nights. Instead of twenty-four artificial light, there may be diurnal natural light. A window view on the world is built into every patient room. Indirect lighting is pleasant. Contemporary colors personify optimism and demonstrate non-hospital attitude. Consideration must be given to unit location and renovations so as to provide easy access. Patients need access to more than higher medical specialization; children need easy access to social and developmental activities in the hospital, and to the outside world.

The transition unit will also be equipped in a fashion to foster normalcy. The environment will be home-like (Olds & Daniel, 1987).

Wooden furniture (chairs, beds) impart a soft appearance in contrast to metal hospital furnishings. We in fact purchased such furniture from a department store. In addition, home furniture such as daybeds provide comfort for guardians wishing to sleep with their child. Cupboards for clothes support the presence of personal items. Storage space should be provided for a personal collection of developmentally appropriate toys. Carpeting will assist soundproofing and provide floor play area. Small televisions on extension arms prevent them from overwhelming a room and annoying other residents and staff. Furnishings will be colorful, bright, matching.

Medical equipment should allow for sufficient monitoring without being the center of unit activities. Simple noninvasive electronic monitoring may be provided on extension arms at ceiling height. These should allow for stepwise removal such as turning off of audio, then cathode ray tube display, then rates, and finally min./max. audio alarms. Telementry should not be used as it would not be used in the home. Noninvasive gas monitoring such as transcutaneous oxygen ($TCpO_2$) and end-tidal CO_2 ($ETCO_2$) should be available for painless evaluation of respiratory status without frequent arterial blood sampling. Unobtrusive hidden wall units for gas and electrical connection are now available. As can be seen, monitoring will be provided similarly to its use in the out-of-hospital long term care environment.

Staffing

We are considering the child with a complex medical condition, often multiple handicaps. Whether medically fragile or technology assisted, the candidate for transition must be stable. Intensive care is replaced by human monitoring and observation. The program goals are discharge planning. Staffing must be multidisciplinary and foster habilitation and enablement.

After discharge, parents or guardians will share care with home health nurses. Nursing is thus the cornerstone of staffing of the pediatric transitional program. Though performing technical procedures, nurses approach the patient and family wholistically. They are the main care providers during hospitalization, assigned twenty-four hours per day. They will provide medical therapies, use medical equipment, monitor patient condition, and record clinical records. As the professionals spending the most time with the child, nurses are essential participants in teaching family and community caretakers. In current parlance, they may even serve as case manager and care coordinator. The most effective are those who transfer from previous experience in intensive care or home care nursing.

The needs of the child dictate the professional components of the interdisciplinary team. Specific medical and developmental status will indicate the need for consultation and ongoing intervention by developmentalists and psychologists as well as physical, occupational, and speech and language therapists. Having been hospitalized, in fact bed bound, for extended periods, intensive therapy by these specialists may be indicated merely for developmental catch up. Specific developmental delay may indicate consultation by developmentalist or educational psychologist. Child Life specialists will address age-appropriate and developmentally oriented play and social interaction. Evaluation and monitoring of family function and resources is the realm of the medical social worker. Stress and coping may indicate the need for ongoing psychological therapy.

Specific medical care must address more than organ system diseases and intercurrent illness. The interplay of pathology, development, and psychosocial aspects highlight the overlap of developmental, behavioral, and rehabilitation pediatrics. These myriad of issues may be covered by one of those subspecialities or by a general pediatrician. Organ-system subspecialists will address their particular medical realms and work together with their medical colleagues. Emphasis, however, must be placed not on membranes or metabolism but rather on management. This can be accomplished by assigned medical direction to a generalist with consultation by subspecialists, or through a co-attending relationship. Having addressed the philosophical and management approach, the assignment of medical direction versus consultation on a particular case or within a particular unit can be determined by local expertise and interest. A pulmonologist sensitive to the nonmedical issues faced by her patient and family and supportive of the roles of the other professionals provides transition comfortably and will be as successful as the generalist who functions as a "chronicologist."

Regional Coordination

Care coordination has been defined as the communication between multiple professionals and the family about their disparate goals so as to carry out a common individualized service plan (Merkens, 1985).

The multiple professionals serving the child and family must function not only as a cast of multiple specialists, but as an interdisciplinary team. Who is involved in the care of the child is determined more by the temperament and approach of the professional than by specialization or credentials. The ability to compromise and to interdigitate care with other professionals is paramount. Respect for the roles of the other professionals and capabilities of other individuals assures coordinated rather than just parallel care. Beyond daily rounds and treatment, weekly team meetings must be participated in by all major professionals. These constructs are native to professionals in psychosocial disciplines but may be foreign to medical specialists. Social science literature suggests that team participation may be an inherent rather than trained skill (Feiger & Schmitt, 1979). Team participants and especially leaders should be chosen based upon interest and these interdisciplinary capabilities.

Coordination is assured by daily function within the unit. No profession can function in isolation. None can assume that their service is so significant or superior as to warrant independent function. Weekly team rounds are the setting to review the care of all current patients. Representatives of all professions and services must participate. Interdisciplinary approach must be fostered.

As the population of children to be served is small, certain steps will assure long-term viability of a pediatric transitional program and unit. These include financing, regionalization and establishment of consortia, involvement of third-party payers, and governmental regulatory reorganization.

Regionalization and centralization of such projects will foster proper utilization (Aday and Andersen, 1988). Inservice education throughout the region will help overcome the expected opposition from other hospitals and doctors. Consortia with tertiary pediatric centers forge relationships of trust with facilities that care for these children during acute phases. Formalized referral through a clearing-house agency, government program, or disease-specific advocacy group will improve acceptance.

A visiting chronic illness transitional consult team will facilitate admission to the program. This team conducts assessments and designs discharge planning for potential patients while still hospitalized in other facilities. After preliminary review of clinical data, the team visits the hospital where the child resides to discuss management and goals and the family's potential for providing home care. Following the visit, the team makes recommendations for appropriate long-term placement possibilities. If indicated, preparation for admission to the transitional unit is carried out by the team. If admitted, the team periodically reports back to the referring medical staff on the patient's progress.

Third party payers must be included in planning for establishment of appropriate rates of payment and to expedite reimbursement for services both in the transitional setting and in the post-hospital setting. Resolution of reimbursement will expedite discharge. Governmental regulatory reorganization must be addressed to allow for coordination of agencies, reimbursement, quality assurance, and removal of barriers to discharge. The health care/child welfare partnership must similarly be established and included in regional planning of the transitional program (Hochstadt & Yost, 1989).

Kohrman (1982) has suggested that a regional transitional program is incomplete without identified custodial facilities qualified to care for children in long term placement. When home placement is not possible or appropriate, skilled nursing facilities are recommended and arranged for so that unit beds can be used for transitional rather than custodial care.

FUNCTION OF THE TRANSITION PROGRAM

The Admission Process

Admission criteria must be devised for use in accurately identifying children who can be served by the program in the special unit, yet to exclude those who are not yet stable enough to safely leave the intensive care unit. Criteria must be firm yet allow for flexibility in application. Their aim is to prevent the inappropriate admission of children who are at risk of sudden decompensation or death. They must be concise for easy understanding by referring physicians and be useable by numerous professions.

Though the use of a ventilator is not standard practice out on the regular ward, a truly unchanging condition may allow altering usual standards with the use of new guidelines with sufficient safeguards. Because there has been extensive experience in the care of ventilator dependent children thoughout the country, this paradigm could be used to demonstrate these new criteria for determination of readiness for discharge from intensive care. Sample criteria are listed in Table 4.2. Similar criteria can be devised for other medical conditions.

Table 4.2. Sample Criteria of Medical Stability: The Child Who Is Ventilator Dependent.

The following criteria have remained unchanged for at least one month, and are foreseen as unchanging indefinitely:
1. Ventilator settings.
2. Blood gases.
3. X-ray of the chest.
4. Pulmonary function tests.
5. Activities of daily living.
6. All other medical conditions.
7. Hospitalization has been continued because of technological care needs (e.g., therapies, treatments, equipment, medications, observation, monitoring) rather than for instability of medical conditions.

Patients are referred to La Rabida's unit from throughout the upper Midwest. Steps of the admission process are outlined in Table 4.3. Admission criteria are reviewed upon referral. If the referring professional remains convinced that their patient meets the criteria and would benefit from transition out of acute hospitalization, the patient is visited in the acute setting. After preliminary screening through discussion, a multidisciplinary team of professionals, called the Chronic Illness Consult Team, makes a group visit to the referring hospital. The team is composed of pediatric chronic illness physician, nurse, social worker, and appropriate therapists. Records are reviewed, the parents are interviewed, and the child is examined. Consensus regarding readiness for transition and transfer to the program is sought. A consultation note is sent to the referring professional, outlining the findings and the decision of the Consult Team visit.

Parents are full participants in the transfer planning process. They are interviewed, consulted, and informed of plans. Their input and consent is sought before commencing transfer and transition. The recent standoff of medical staff by armed parents in a Chicago P.I.C.U. was apparently forced by differences in goals for their child which were perceived but not adopted by the hospital. The parents legal rights for determining outcome in that case have been recognized; parents' ethical rights for determination must also be recognized.

Table 4.3. Chronology of Admission of the Transitional Care Unit.

Referral
Review of admission criteria
Review of patient medical records
Visit by Chronic Illness Consult Team
Acceptance for admission
Parental participation and consent
Development of discharge criteria
Transfer/admit to Transitional Unit

Table 4.4. Steps in Transitioning the Child with Chronic Illness.

Medical stabilization
Realignment of care schedules and procedures
Readjustment of monitoring
Transfer to portable and long term equipment
Identification of community providers
Arrangement of financial resources
Training of home and community providers
Organization of community-based services
Preparation of discharge manual
Discharge

It is imperative to establish discharge criteria prior to commencement of transitional programming, especially prior to admission to the free standing unit. By stating discharge criteria at the outset, all interested participants and observers are aware of the service goals for that patient. Progress can be gauged and next steps planned for. Misunderstanding and manipulation can be minimized, and progress maximized.

Transitioning

All activities in the transitional care unit are focused on discharge planning. Medical care is readjusted to reflect a regimen to be used out of hospital. Home care equipment is acquired. Funding for home care is secured. Community-based services are arranged. Home care and community providers are taught care of the child. (Table 4.4.)

The staff of the transitional unit knows home care procedures. They can readjust treatment protocols from acute to longterm. Noninvasive laboratory testing is used. Monitoring is decreased in frequency and shifted to visual from electronic. New protocols can be tested in the safety of the unit. With these steps the child and parents can become accustomed to new protocols in a safe controlled environment.

The entire team of providers meets weekly to review and update daily care and goals for discharge. All relevant and pertinent subject areas are addressed. These include but are not limited to medical, nursing, development, psychology, education, social, child life. All professionals providing care attend. Each reports on progress within their realm. Then open discussion is fashioned to shape a consensus on goals for the next week and longterm.

Daily rounds, sessions, treatments and therapies are held according to usual schedules. In the transition unit, however, they are done as they will be in the home. Even medical procedures can be done in the crib or on the floor. After morning care, the bed is pushed aside and the child is taken out for developmentally appropriate activities. Infants and toddlers are placed on the rugged floors for crawling and play. Preschoolers and school children leave the unit to attend classroom programming whenever possible.

After lunch lights are dimmed for nap time. Children with respiratory conditions and cardiac defects consume extra calories by their condition, so extra rest is necessary for recuperation and growth. All activities are scheduled around normal biologic, family, and privacy activities.

Care takers become teachers in the transitional unit. Parents are taught steps of care whenever they are present. Daybeds, closets, and private bathrooms provide an environment for them to sleep over and increasingly assume care around the clock. Parents can truly become the specialist on their own child through learning and doing all care from physical therapy, to nursing care to developmental stimulation.

Special intensive teaching days for community providers are scheduled toward the end of hospitalization in the transition unit. These pack in didactic lectures and hands-on demonstrations at the bedside. Effective scheduling will assure that teaching from all involved professionals will cover all needed care realms. By the time of discharge, the community providers will be prepared to assume all aspects of care of the transitioned child.

A discharge manual covering all instructional units and guidelines as per the assessed needs is assembled for each child. This manual is the outline and reference for training and care. Each procedure must be outlined, and policies and contingency plans are also addressed. This manual can be read by providers-in-training at their own convenience, used during teaching, and referenced later (Aitken, 1988).

As discharge approaches, the parents and community providers may try a dry run of long term care. In the safety of the transition unit, home providers deliver all care, but may ask for assistance. This trial is most effective if realistic—parents providing care, phoning out for consultation, ordering equipment—for a week. They may obtain meals in the cafeteria, but reside with their child in a private room without scheduled care by hospital staff. Staff may visit socially during breaks. Hospital staff intervene only for emergencies. By the end of the trial period the community providers and parents will have demonstrated their skills to the unit staff and affirmed their own self confidence.

The child is ready for discharge from the transition unit.

TRANSITIONING THE CHILD WELFARE CLIENT

The health care/child welfare partnership is a paradigm of interagency coordination and interprofessional service provision (Hochstadt & Yost, 1989). Health care professionals must accept the ascendance, even precedence, of nonmedical issues. Delays and dealings with other professionals will tax health professionals' morale. Child welfare professionals will have to work in the stressful, seemingly mythical, world of high tech medicine. Identification and training of foster parents differentiates this partnership from the discharge of children to birth parents.

The health care/child welfare partnership is melded when health care workers refer a child to the child welfare agencies. Medical care takers will refer a family when the constellation reveals gaps in family strength placing the child at risk for neglect or maltreatment. Or the child welfare services may have already been added to the service cadre because the original condition was caused or exacerbated by abuse or neglect. The transitional program will be the source of discharge planning but will have the added obligation of creating a strong home environment or arranging custodial care.

It can no longer be assumed that every biologic parent will chose to care for their child in the family home. The perception that children with technology dependency and medically fragility could be cared for by lay persons outside the hospital was the philosophical frontier a decade ago. Contemporary philosophical issues include informing parents of the risk and benefits of options for care for their child and accepting their choice. The burdens of home care such as cost, stress, disruption, loss of privacy, and loss of freedom must be considered by the informed parents. Even potential guilt over death occurring under their care must be explained and assimilated by the parents. Some families may find these burdens too onerous or be deemed unable to assume them. Families should not be "forced" to take their child home or made to feel that they are "bad parents" if they are unable to do so. Custodial placement or some other alternative through social welfare must then be utilized.

Medical personnel may come to be concerned about a particular family's ability to provide care for their child in the home. Child welfare professionals must be consulted to assist in the evaluation of such a family. The health care and child welfare professionals must communicate about the realities of medical care of the child, the family's assets, and the roles of health and welfare service systems.

Foster home placement may be determined to be the best alternative to home placement with the biologic parents. The identification of capable and interested foster families is carried out by the welfare agency. But foster placement will necessitate the teaching of caretaking to foster parents by medical professionals.

Specialized training about the generic issues generated by children with severe chronic illness will impart information about care of the child and serve to reduce apprehension associated with this responsibility. Training specific to the care of each child is presented "at the bedside" in the transitional unit by the transitional care team. Transitional program philosophy and physical environment welcomes biologic, foster and agency family members into the facility, and invites their assumption of direct care. The child is progressively transitioned from hospital to community.

SUMMARY

More children with severe chronic illnesses are surviving. Many are dependent upon modern technology to survive, or are medically fragile. Our society has adopted a philosophy of deinstitutionalization and mainstreaming. Children not saved two decades ago, who were perhaps institutionalized a decade ago, are now sent home or to the best alternative residential setting. They survive and their familes cope through strong support. Transition from P.I.C.U. to home or best alternative is a labor-intensive process. Transition Team, program, and unit provide the care and planning for that change. The health care/child welfare alliance must function to shift care of the child from hospital to his/her family, foster care, or long term residential placement.

REFERENCES

Aday, L. A. & Andersen, R. M. (1988). *Lessons and implications from the VACPEP Study.* In L. A. Aday, M. J. Aitken, & D. H. Wegner (Ed.), *Pediatric Home Care* (pp. 323–332). Chicago, IL: Pluribus Press, Inc.

Aitken, M. J. (1988). *What kinds of programs emerged?* In L. A. Aday, M. J. Aitken, & D. H. Wegner (Ed.), *Pediatric Home Care* (pp. 95–156). Chicago, IL: Pluribus Press, Inc.

Brewer, E. J., McPherson, M., Magrab, P. R., & Hutchins V. L. (1989). *Family-centered, community-based, coordinated care for children with special health care needs. Pediatrics, 83* (6), 1055–1060.

Feiger, S. & Schmitt, M. H. (1979). *Collegiality and interdisciplinary teams: It's measurement and its effects. Social Science and Medicine, 13a*, 217–229.

Hochstadt, N. J., & Yost, D. M. (1989). *The health care-child welfare partnership: Transitioning medically complex children to the community. Children's Health Care, 18* (1), 4–11.

Kohrman, A. F. (1982). Alternatives for care of ventilator dependent children. Surgeon General's Conference on Children with Handicaps and Their Families. Philadelphia, December, 1982.

La Rabida Children's Hospital and Research Center (1984). *Sending the ventilator-dependent children home: the chronic illness transitional care program.*

Merkens, M. (1984). *Transitional care for chronically ill children.* Unpublished manuscript, La Rabida Children's Hospital, Chicago.

Merkens, M. (1985). *Communication and coordination.* In M. J. Merkens, C. K. Burr, & J. M. Perrin (Ed.), Primary Providers in the Care of Handicapped Children: Conference Report (pp. 23–26). Nashville, TN: Vanderbilt University.

Merkens, M. (1990). *A pediatric chronic illness transitional care unit. Children's Health Care, 19*, 4–9.

Merkens, M. & Anderson, P. (1983). A pediatric transitional care program and clinical consult team. Workshop, Association for Care of Children's Health (ACCH).

Office of Technology Assessment. (1987). Technology-dependent children: Hospital v. Home Care—A technical memorandum, OTA-TM-H-38. Washington, D.C.: U.S. Government Printing Office.

Okamato, G. A. & Shurtleff, D. B. (1981). Perceived first contact care for disabled children. *Pediatrics, 67*, 530–535.

Olds, A. & Daniel, P. (1987). Child Health Care Facilities: Design Guidelines-Literature Outline. Washington, D.C.: Association for the Care o Children's Health (ACCH).

Perrin, J. M., Merkens, M. J., & Kohrman, A. F. (1983). Regionalization for chronically ill children: Can it be done? Workshop, Ambulatory Pediatric Association (APA).

Pollack, M. M., Wilkinson, J. D., & Glass, N. L. (1987). Long-stay pediatric intensive care unit patients: Outcome and resource utilization. *Pediatrics, 80*, 855–860.

Section III

Discharge Planning:
The Link to the Community

CHAPTER 5

THE NURSE'S ROLE: DISCHARGING SPECIAL NEEDS CHILDREN TO FOSTER CARE

SUSAN SULLIVAN-BOLYAI

INTRODUCTION

Ten to 15% of our nation's children under 18 years of age have a chronic health impairment (Hobbs & Perrin, 1985; Hobbs, Perrin & Ireys, 1985). Due to the many advances in medical technology and treatment, more children are surviving the effects of prematurity, congenital anomalies and childhood trauma (Office of Technology Assessment, 1987; Gliedman & Roth, 1980). As a result, there is a growing need for professional nurses with strong backgrounds in discharge planning and continuity of care to work with these children and their families.

Many of these special needs children reside for long periods of time in hospitals. Some of them, due to complex social situations, end up as wards of the state requiring temporary or long-term foster placement (Hochstadt & Yost, 1989). For these children, the professional nurse plays an integral role in developing a comprehensive continuity of care plan, including a hospital discharge plan.

The purpose of this chapter is to describe the nurse's role in the comprehensive discharge planning process necessary to effectively and safely transition medically complex children from the hospital into a specialized foster home. This chapter will cover the assessment process, development of a teaching plan, training the foster family, developing the follow-up plan, the evaluation process, and other tasks required to discharge a child to a specialized foster home.

THE NURSING ASSESSMENT

Once child welfare professionals have identified a family that is committed to fostering a child with special needs, and is motivated to learn the necessary care, a comprehensive nursing assessment of the prospective parents must be completed. This assessment determines the knowledge and experience base of the foster parents. Learning readiness and ability must also be assessed (Smith, 1987; Voland, 1988). This provides the nurse with baseline information from which to develop a teaching plan, assess any misinformation that may have been communicated and clarify any misunderstandings that the foster parents may have (Smith, 1988; McClelland, Kelly & Buckwaiter, 1985). Misperceptions should be clarified immediately and communicated to the rest of the health care team. Reinforcement of correct information should become part of the training plan as well.

Prior to the first training session the family's level of interest, attentiveness, and appropriateness of inquiries should be assessed. Occasionally, a foster family may be very eager to learn the child's care but their interest may wane. This may be the result of fears and/ or a developing awareness of the complexity of the child's needs. If this occurs, support and counselling should be provided by both nursing and social work staff. At the same time the sensitive issue of whether to continue training and placement with the family, or to cancel the plan, must be dealt with. The foster parents should be given sufficient time to integrate all of the information needed to make this decision and, with non-judgemental support, arrive at a mutually agreed upon decision.

Another step in the assessment process is the determination of the foster family's ability to learn the child's care (Johnson, Giovannoni & Driscoll, 1986). This, as with readiness, should be screened prior to the placement commitment. The nurse must assess any perceptual limitations such as deficits in reading ability, sight, hearing, language problems, and fine motor limitations that might interfere with technical care. All of these data must be gathered prior to developing an appropriate individualized teaching plan. Often, asking the foster parents how they learn best elicits important information about their learning style. This will assist the nurse in developing an appropriate training plan.

Often it is crucial that there be more than one person in the household be capable of caring for the medically complex child. This ad-

Table 5.1. Needs Assessment.

Home Environment	Yes	No	Community Access	Yes	No
Smoke detector			Fire education		
Fire extinguisher			Paramedic service		
Adequate electrical service/ outlets			E.R. service		
Working phone			Local pediatrician		
Heat			Pharmacy access		
Running water			Respite care		
Refrigerator			Public transportation		
Physical facility to accommodate disability:			Nutrition service		
Ramp			Day care for disabled		
Accessible bathroom (if child requires private duty nurse in home) a minimum area of 9×9 ft will be required			Developmental/educational programs including speech, occupational, physical therapies, infant development		
Storage space for equipment and supplies					

Equipment Needs	Yes	No	Support Systems	Yes	No
Wheelchair			Alternative caregiver(s)		
Stroller			Emergency caregiver		
Car seat			Emergency transportation		
High chair			Homemaker service		
Feeder seat			Home therapy		
Bath chair			Home nursing service		
Respiratory equipment					
Nutritional equipment					
Equipment company referral					

NOTE: Adapted from *The family as care manager: Home care coordination for medically fragile children* (p. 3–5) by J. Kaufman and K. Lichtenstein, 1985, Washington, D.C.: United States Department of Maternal Child Health.

ditional support provides for such contingencies as emergency room visits, clinic visits, shopping, social events, respite care, and fluctuating work schedules. As a result, each family member who will be caring for the child in the home must be part of the assessment.

Finally, a comprehensive nursing needs assessment should include an evaluation of the home environment. This assessment should include the home safety and the capacity of the physical environment to sustain the discharge plan. The assessment should also look at the foster parents' willingness to utilize community resources. Table 5.1 provides guidelines for assessing the home environment.

THE TEACHING PLAN

Training Content

The professional nurse's role in parent education is threefold. The
nurse is responsible for identifying the appropriate training content
to be taught to the foster parents, educating the family about the
child's medical condition and associated problems, as well as instructing the parents in the technical nursing care of the child.

The professional nurse's role in teaching technical skills may vary.
For example, some hospitals have large respiratory therapy departments that may assist in some of the technical respiratory training
such as chest suctioning, administering nebulization treatments, and
ventilator management. This may attenuate the nurse's role. On the
other hand, the nurse may be directly responsible for instructing the
family in such techniques as tracheostomy care, gastrostomy care,
administration of medications, cardiopulmonary resuscitation, physical assessment, including signs and symptoms of potential medical
problems, and solving routine medical and nursing care issues.

Rehabilitation needs of the child such as positioning, turning, range
of motion, oral feeding techniques, and developmental stimulation
may be demonstrated by the appropriate health care providers with
reinforcement by the nurse.

The nurse also has an important role in educating the family about
well child care and preventive care issues such as immunizations,
child safety, parent-child relationships, facilitating appropriate growth
and development and positive behavioral management techniques.

A formalized teaching plan should be developed by the nurse trainer.
The plan should be guided by mutually agreed upon trainee-trainer
goals and objectives. To assist the nurse trainer in developing an
individualized teaching plan, standardized discharge objectives have
been developed (Sullivan-Bolyai, 1990). This plan includes well child
care, general respiratory care, tracheostomy, naso-gastric/gastros-
tomy tube, and ventilator care. Generally, the teaching plan is flexible
so that objectives can be added or deleted to enable the plan to be
individualized for each trainee. All objectives must be accomplished
by the designated trainer before home passes or discharge can take
place. Multiple copies of the plan provide documentation for the
medical chart, the discharge planner, the parents and home care
agencies. Foster families can share this plan with other health professionals and with their child welfare agency as proof of proficiency.

Guidelines for training in some areas such as tracheostomy and gastrostomy care have already been developed (Sullivan-Bolyai, 1990). Having standardized guidelines is helpful in developing a consistent approach to training given that multiple trainers may be involved. The professional nurse plays an active role in the discharge training process whether teaching the family directly, or coordinating these activities with other members of the health care team.

Teaching Materials

An array of audio-visual aids and reading materials are available to assist trainers in educating foster families (Smith, 1987, Ahmann, 1986; Association for the Care of Children's Health, 1987, 1988). It is helpful for the nurse to utilize teaching dolls equipped with medical assisted devices such as tracheostomy and gastrostomy tubes, ventriculoperitoneal shunts, and central lines (Patient Puppets, 1986).

Accommodations should be made for those individuals who may not read or speak English; for these individuals multi-lingual teaching aids are essential. Teaching techniques and aids for those who are illiterate must also be made available to the trainer (Doak, Doak & Root, 1985). Generally, the trainer moves slowly from videotapes and trainee observation to doll demonstration, to "hands-on" experience. This enables the trainees to gain confidence and command of the required skills.

When written materials are used, it is generally best to gear the text no higher than a sixth grade level (Smith, 1987). It is helpful to provide the foster family with a loose leaf binder to store all written handouts they acquire from various health care disciplines. This binder may include such information as a medical summary, articles regarding the medical diagnosis, specific nursing discharge orders, an outline of the child's "typical day," guidelines for meeting the developmental needs of the child, nutritional information, information regarding medications (i.e., dosage, frequency of administration, side effects, storage, etc.), instructions as to when to call the doctor, public service company phone numbers (i.e., Fire Department and Paramedics), nursing agency and equipment company phone numbers, an emergency room letter, and a copy of the home equipment list. Each binder can be individualized to meet the needs of the particular child and family.

Parent-Staff Training Schedules

Once the foster parents have agreed to learn the child's care a training schedule should be set-up by nursing. Having multiple copies of this schedule is very helpful. The training schedule should include the dates, times, and the name of the trainer. In addition to the foster family having a copy of this schedule all relevant hospital personnel should be familiar with the schedule. Training schedules often have to be adjusted to conform to the learning "styles" and schedules of the foster family. The training schedule may also be used to keep track of those appointments that are kept and those that are not. This information may be useful to discern a pattern of ambivalence regarding the continuation of the training program by the parents.

IMPLEMENTATION

Training Time Frame

It is often difficult to determine the exact number of training hours needed for a foster parent to become competent and comfortable in caring for a child with special needs. Each individual learns at a different pace. Learning is dependent upon the individual's previous knowledge and experience, readiness, willingness to participate in the training, ability, and comfort level with the child; as well as the child's comfort level with the trainees (Smith, 1987). Equally as important, is the type of tasks and skills needed to be acquired. For example, an experienced and competent foster mother planning to care for a child with bronchopulmonary dysplasia, who will be receiving only nebulization treatments, may be able to learn the child's care in one session. Of course, several pre-placement visits are encouraged to help the child and foster parents adjust to each other. On the other hand, the training time needed for children requiring more extensive nursing care is harder to predict. For example, Chadderdon and Johnson (1986) note that motivated foster parents having only minor anxiety around tracheostomy care, may complete training in approximately 6 to 8 sessions (2 to 3 hours per session). Flexibility must be built into the scheduling to allow for differences in learning speed and comfort level with the child's care. It is often helpful for the health professional to reflect on their own educational and training experiences to understand how difficult it is for foster families to feel comfortable and competent in caring for children with complex medical needs.

At times, foster parents may complete the necessary training prior to state approval of home care funding. This can be a frustrating time for the foster parents, the child and the staff. Identifying this potential problem for foster parents early in the discharge process, and providing an understanding of the complex bureaucratic processes involved in home care funding, may alleviate some of the angry or frustrating feelings that foster parents often experience in such a situation.

Other Training Suggestions

During hospital based-training, it is advisable to have a maximum of two consistent nurse staff members serve as trainers. This reduces fragmentation of the educational process. Ideally, one nurse on the day shift and one nurse on the afternoon/evening shift can accommodate the foster parents' work and/or family schedules. One nurse should be assigned the responsibility of coordinating the training with members of the other health care disciplines. If the foster parents cannot attend the training sessions during daytime hours, special arrangements may need to be made so that all members of the health care team working with the child have an opportunity to meet with the foster parents.

EVALUATION

Evaluation of the training program should be an ongoing process (Smith, 1987). Regular meetings should be scheduled between the foster parents and the trainers to discuss training progress, parental feelings about the training program, frustrations, fears, questions regarding any aspects of the teaching plan, or other modifications of the plan that may enhance the training process.

Time Limits

Occasionally, even after a comprehensive multidisciplinary assessment and planning process, problems may arise. For example, the parents may be unable to grasp fine motor mechanics of some of the essential skills required to safely care for the child. If this occurs, further evaluation of the parents will be needed. Different teaching methods and/or tools may need to be utilized. At different times, the foster parents may be too anxious or fearful to reach competence in the requisite skill. Methods to decrease the anxiety level should be explored. A revised time frame, to decrease the foster parents' anxiety level, should be considered.

Another potential problem requiring ongoing evaluation is attendance. Sporadically kept appointments can be a sign of anxiety or could be related to the foster parents' ambivalence about the placement. Ongoing evaluation and periodic meetings with the foster parents and the child welfare professionals, may be necessary to identify problems and develop alternative solutions. It is advisable, at the outset of training, to set a limit on the number of missed sessions. The consequences of the foster parents' failure to keep training appointments should be discussed early.

Assessing Clinical Competence

Once the foster parents have successfully demonstrated the required care techniques and have completed all components of the training plan, they are ready to move on to the next phase. It is often useful to schedule an "overnight pass" in the hospital once the formal training has been completed. By staying overnight in the hospital, and being responsible for all of the child's care with minimal nursing involvement, the foster parents are able to try out their newly acquired skills in a safe environment. This provides the nursing staff with an opportunity to evaluate their clinical competence. This is often a useful stepping stone to the next training phase—the overnight home pass.

OTHER NURSING DISCHARGE RESPONSIBILITIES

Development of an Equipment List

Development of a comprehensive equipment list should be started early in the discharge planning process. There are a variety of standardized, and purchaseable, institutional equipment checklists available (Children's Hospital Medical Center, 1988; Children's Memorial Hospital, 1989 and La Rabida Children's Hospital, 1985). Another option is for the discharge planning team to collaborate with a designated home health care agency and vendor to develop a standardized institutional checklist of their own. An equipment list will aid the foster family, and the discharge planning nurses, to determine the specific equipment and supplies needed for home care. At times, the amount of equipment and supplies needed in the home may vary from what was needed in the hospital. This results from the different techniques often used in the hospital and home care. For example, a clean technique is used for tracheostomy care in the home while a sterile technique is used in the hospital. As a result, the Shiley tracheostomy tube is changed approximately one time per week in the home as opposed to two times per week in the hospital.

Ordering Equipment

It is very helpful for the foster family to be part of the decision making process when choosing home care resources such as equipment vendors. The relationship between equipment vendors and the foster family is a crucial one. Initially, the hospital may provide the foster family with a developed list of approved equipment vendors from which they may choose (O'Hare & Terry, 1988). If time allows, the family may wish to interview several local vendor representatives. Nursing can also provide the family with a list of questions they may wish to ask vendors.

Prior to discharge the family should be given a copy of the monthly supply list for home care products. This will encourage a continuity of care between the equipment vendor and the family.

Home Health Agency Referral

There are several types of home nursing support that can be offered to foster families depending upon the complexity of the foster child's medical condition. Children with specialized care needs such as a tracheostomy or a ventilator can usually qualify for private duty nursing in the home. A nurse provides for the child's care during the scheduled work hours in the home. In many states the federal Medicaid Waiver Program determines the number of home nursing hours each child can receive. Respite hours may also be included in this type of agreement.

Another type of home nursing support available to foster families is the intermittent visit. In this arrangement the home health agency provides professional nursing care to the home several times per week. The nurse is available to monitor treatments, medications, nutritional support, the child's physical and emotional development, and provide emotional support to the foster parents. The duration of these services varies from state to state depending on funding availability.

As with the selection of equipment vendors, the foster parents should also be consulted as to the choice of the home nursing agency. Here again, it is helpful for the nurse discharge planner to supply the foster parents with a list of questions to ask the home health agency representative.

Occasionally, home health aides and/or homemaker services may be available to assist in the child's daily care or to free-up the foster parents for household chores so that they can better care for the child. Again, payment for such services will vary from state to state and from insurer to insurer.

Home Health Staff Orientation

Prior to the child's discharge to home care, an orientation for the home health care staff should be set up by the hospital's nursing discharge planner to provide them with as much background and technical information as possible. The amount of time alloted for this will vary depending on the child's condition. For example, a one day didactic and clinical orientation for the home health nurses is suggested several days prior to discharge for children going home with a tracheostomy. In order to limit liability, and for quality assurance purposes, it is important for hospital nursing staff to verify the credentials (i.e., licenses) and competence (i.e., cardiopulmonary resuscitation, pediatric clinical experience, pediatric tracheostomy training) of home health nurses. As part of the home health staff orientation, summaries of the care provided by *all* specialties should be given to the home care staff. Prior to discharge, home health care staff should also participate in the child's care under the supervision of the primary nurse. A final discharge staffing involving the home health care personnel, hospital staff, funding agencies, the foster family and the child welfare agency should be held the week prior to discharge. Final changes and/or modifications of the discharge plan can be made at that time. This also provides all members of the hospital based team and the home health care team to resolve any last minute issues.

Preparing Foster Parents for In-Home Health Personnel

It is important to prepare the foster family for working with nursing and other health care personnel in their home. The best source of such information comes from other parents who have successfully worked with home health care providers. Having a predetermined list of foster parents who have agreed to talk with new families prior to discharge can be very effective. Parent support groups or informal hospital based parent coffee hours can be very helpful to new foster families. These groups permit parents to interact with one another, share experiences and solve problems related to home health care issues. At times, the emotional support provided by these groups can be invaluable. SKIP (Sick Kids Need Involved People) is a parent support group having chapters throughout the country. This group provides support, as well as information on resources and child advocacy (Sick Kids Need Involved People, 1982). There are also some audiovisual aids available to assist families caring for medically complex children (Illinois Division of Services for Crippled Children, 1988). Lastly, prior to discharge the nurse-trainer or discharge planner should discuss with the foster family issues such as scheduling, setting rules in the home for home health care personnel, employee-employer relationships, confidentiality and liability (Kaufman & Lichtenstein, 1985; Rose & Thomas, 1987).

Sharing Information

Prior to the child's discharge it is essential to set up a communication network between the foster parents, the hospital, the medical follow-up facility, and community agencies. A consistent contact person should be identified for the family to serve as liaison (case manager) amongst all of the above resources. The frequency and method of communication also should be determined prior to discharge. This important case management function will be discussed in greater detail later in this chapter.

Other Community Issues

There are other discharge planning tasks, not directly related to nursing care, that the professional nurse may be responsible for organizing. This may include the child's rehabilitation needs in the community, nutritional care, notification of public service and utility companies prior to discharge, assurance that the appropriate medical information is documented and available for home/community use, identification and coordination of medical follow-up and educational/school services.

If the child requires in-home therapies (e.g., respiratory therapy, physical therapy) the nurse may also assist in identifying quality home care agencies that provide these services and may also make the initial referral.

The child's nutritional home care needs should not be overlooked at discharge. The professional nurse may identify, in conjunction with a registered dietitian, specific dietary recommendations. Nutritional support may be supplied through a combination of equipment vendors and programs (e.g., the Women, Infant and Children Program—WIC, the Social Security Disability Program). Foster parents should be provided with techniques to access nutritional support on an ongoing basis so that there is no interruption of services in the transition to home care.

An essential step in the discharge process is the notification of public service and utility companies of the child's impending discharge. The professional nurse may coordinate the sending of letters to the family's local paramedic/fire department, electric company, gas company, and phone company alerting them of the discharge date. Letters to these public services should alert them to the specific requirements of the child should there be a disruption of service (e.g., due to bad weather or other natural causes). Specific instructions for the paramedics or fire department should also be included in the letter. The foster family should also be provided with a list of emergency phone numbers for these public services. Some families have given a copy of this list to neighbors as an additional safety measure.

Prior to discharge the nurse should be sure that the child's physician has prepared a letter describing the child's basic medical condition, baseline data, current treatment plan, medication regime, names and phone numbers of medical staff at the hospital. This letter is invaluable if the child must be taken to an emergency room or other medical facility unfamiliar with the child's care. Copies of this letter should be given to each of the caregivers including home health care personnel. This letter should be updated periodically.

Finding local medical care for foster chidren with complex medical needs is often challenging. It is often helpful to develop a list of local pediatricians willing to care for a medically complex child. Prior to discharge, the foster family and the hospital based physician, should determine where the child will receive the most efficacious follow-up medical care. Often, a general pediatrician in the community can provide most of the well child follow-up care while other physicians may provide the speciality care required by the child. Every effort should be made to obtain as many services in close proximity to the foster parents' home.

If the child is of school age, and is going to a new school setting due to the foster home placement, it is essential to clarify what services the child will need in the classroom. The nurse can help develop special care guidelines needed by the school nurse to manage the child in the classroom. This task should be done in collaboration with the school staff prior to discharge. Often, equipment and supplies will be needed by the school. As a result, extra supplies will have to be ordered before the child can begin school. If at all possible the school nurse should attend the final discharge conference to assist in the development of the school plan.

Home Passes Prior to Discharge

Home passes are an important part of the discharge process—for the child as well as the foster parents. If the child is medically stable, and the foster parents are trained and comfortable with the child's care, home passes can be arranged by the nurse according to the parents' work and/or home schedule. These passes provide valuable trial and error experience in a controlled manner. If modifications of the home care plan are needed this can then be accomplished prior to the formal discharge.

Initially, a 4 to 6 hour pass is suggested. All the equipment and supplies must be delivered to the home, set-up, and reviewed by the vendor prior to the pass. If this initial pass is successful the length of subsequent passes can be increased; the foster parents' comfort level is a useful guide in determining how rapidly the length of passes can be extended. Depending on the foster parents' wishes, the 24 hour overnight pass may include the home health nurse(s) working several shifts that day, making a single home visit or the parents may wish to "solo." The phone numbers of key hospital personnel are given to the family so they may call with specific questions or just for support. The child and the family return to the hospital the next day to review the previous day's events. If there were no problems and the family felt comfortable with the process, and the child remained medically stable, the formal discharge can take place.

Continuity of Care

Setting up a continuity of care system for each child with special needs is another important part of the nursing discharge planning process. Continuity of care is defined as a coordinated, ongoing process of activities, involving the child, family and the interdisciplinary health providers, working together to facilitate the transition between the health care facility and home (Thomas, Wicks, & Gregory, 1986). This process encourages timely and accurate communication amongst team members, the coordination of services, and the involvement of the family in the decision making process. An effective continuity of care program assists the payers, providers of care, and the consumers to maximize their resources, and ensures that quality care is received while redundant services are eliminated. Generally, an effective continuity of care program relies on the designation of a health care professional to serve as a case manager. In some instances, the family may choose to do their own case management. Many continuity of care programs utilize a professional nurse as the case manager (see Table 5.2). Developing a continuity of care system, with a designated case manager, prior to discharge completes the comprehensive plan necessary to provide quality care for medically complex children.

COST EFFECTIVENESS AND QUALITY ASSURANCE

The key to the entire discharge planning process is the guarantee of quality care delivered in a cost effective manner. The professional nurse plays an essential role in the quality assurance process. The nurse may assess the foster parents' satisfaction (formally or informally) with the discharge process and with the home care plan. It is essential for nurses to gather information about the satisfaction and effectiveness of the discharge planning process so that other foster parents and children going through the same process will benefit from previous experience. This information assists the professional nurse to continually monitor the effectiveness of the program.

Table 5.2. The Nurse's Role in Continuity of Care.

Components of Continuity of Care	Role/Tasks of Care Manager
Community Based Care: This component includes ensuring that medical follow-up, home care (incl. equipment, supplies, intermittent or private duty nursing care, home health aide, homemaker, therapy services, nutritional needs), school and any other community based services are identified, utilized and evaluated for the child and family on an ongoing basis.	*Assessment* —Ongoing child/family assessment of health care and associated needs —Preadmission assessment —Predischarge assessment —Community resource identification (inc. financial) —Telephone triage
Effective Pre-Admission Activities: This includes the scheduling of needed hospital services, notification to disciplines of child's equipment, medical, nursing, emotional, developmental, educational and nutritional needs, as well as the parent's educational and emotional needs prior to hospitalization. Information is collected by the case manager from community-based services and distributed to appropriate hospital staff.	*Plan* —Development of child/family care plan and ongoing evaluation and modification —Determine admission *Implementation* —Facilitate acquisition of services/ community resources —Monitor services/community resources (phone/home visits)
Admission to the Hospital: This should include comprehensive interdisciplinary assessment of child and family needs, as well as a discharge plan identified. The case manager ensures all assessments are completed and a discharge plan is in place.	—Facilitate/coordinate discharge plan —Parent-child education —Physician-family liaison (interpreter intermediary) *Evaluation*
Hospital Stay: This should be family focused with the case manager or identified resource person coordinating staffings and/or services needed with hospital staff.	—Evaluate discharge plan —Continuous evaluation of services: medical, nursing, community, financial
Discharge Planning: An interdisciplinary team effort is mandatory to create and implement a comprehensive plan for returning the child to a safe environment in the community.	
Follow-up: Ongoing data collection regarding the child's physical, emotional, and future health care needs should be monitored. This may include home and clinic visits.	

NOTE: Adapted from *The first national task force for pediatric continuity of care* by R. Thomas, K. Wicks, and D. Gregory 1986, unpublished manuscript.

SUMMARY

A great deal of preparation must occur before a medically complex child can safely be discharged to foster care. The professional nurse may play many roles in this process. As a discharge planner, teacher/ trainer, advocate, and resource person the nurse, along with other members of the hospital based health care team, helps to develop a safe and cost effective transition to community care. The ultimate goal is to provide the medically complex child with an effective transition from the hospital to a well trained and caring foster home in the community.

REFERENCES

Ahmann, E. (1986). *Home care for high risk infants*. Maryland: Aspen Press.

Association for the Care of Children's Health. (1988). *Bibliography for parent education materials*. Washington, DC.

Association for the Care of Children's Health. (1987). *Family centered care for children with special health care needs*. Washington, DC.

Chadderdon, C. & Johnson, D. (1986). Teaching the patient and family about home care. In D. Johnson, R. Giovannoni & S. Driscoll (Eds.), *Ventilator Assisted Patient Care* (pp. 107–153). Maryland: Aspen Press.

Children's Hospital National Medical Center. (1988). *Continuity of care/discharge planning reference notebook*. (Available from [Children's Hospital National Medical Center, III Michigan Avenue, N.W., Washington, D.C. 20010]).

Children's Memorial Hospital. (1985). *Discharge planning guidelines*. (Available from [Discharge Planning Department, Children's Memorial Hospital, 2300 Children's Plaza, Chicago, IL 60614]).

Gliedman, J. & Roth, W. (1980). *The unexpected minority: Handicapped children in America*. New York: Harcourt, Brace & Jovanovic.

Hobbs, N. & Perrin, J (1985). *Issues in the care of children with chronic illness*. San Francisco: Jossey-Bass.

Hobbs, N., Perrin, J. & Ireys, H. T. (1985). *Chronically ill children and their families*. San Francisco: Jossey-Bass.

Hochstadt, N. J. & Yost, D. M. (1989). The health care-child welfare partnership: Transitioning medically complex children to the community. *Children's Health Care, 18*, 4–12.

Illinois Division of Services for Crippled Children. (1988). *Home care videotape series* [Video cassette]. Evanston, IL: Medical Educational Services, Inc.

Johnson, D., Giovannoni, R. & Driscoll, S. (1986). *Ventilator-assisted patient care planning for hospital discharge and home care.* Maryland: Aspen Press.

Kaufman, J. & Lichtenstein, K. (1985). *The family as care manager: Home care coordination for medically fragile children.* Washington, DC: The U.S. Department of Maternal and Child Health.

La Rabida Children's Hospital and Research Center. (1985). *Institutional equipment checklist.* Chicago, IL: Author.

McClelland, E., Kelly, K. & Buckwaiter, K. (1985). *Continuity of care: Advancing the concept of discharge planning.* Florida: Grune & Stratton.

Office of Technology Assessment (1987). Technology-dependent children: Hospital v. home care—A technical memorandum (U.S. Congress, No. OTA-TM-H-38). Washington, D.C.: U.S. Government Printing Office.

O'Hare, P. & Terry, M. (1988). *Discharge planning: Strategies for assuring continuity of care.* Maryland: Aspen Press.

Patient puppets (manufacturer). (1986). Available from [Patient Puppets, 40 Home Street, Winnipeg, Manitoba, R3G, Canada]).

Rose, M. & Thomas, R. (1987). *Children with chronic conditions.* Florida: Grune & Stratton.

Sick kids need involved people. (1982). (Available from [Sick Kids Need Involved People—a parent support group, 216 Newport Drive, Severna Park, Maryland 21146]).

Smith, C. (Ed.). (1987). *Patient education: Nurses in partnership with other health professionals.* Florida: Grune & Stratton.

Sullivan-Bolyai, S. (1990). *Continuity of care manual.* (Available from [Nursing Department, La Rabida Children's Hospital and Research Center, East 65th Street at Lake Michigan, Chicago, IL. 60649]).

Thomas, R., Wicks, K. & Gregory, D. (1986). *The first national task force for pediatric continuity of care.* Unpublished manuscript.

Volland, P. (1988). *Discharge planning: An interdisciplinary approach to continuity of care.* Maryland: National Health Publishing.

Section IV
Psychosocial Issues

CHAPTER 6

THE ROLE OF SOCIAL SERVICES IN THE PLACEMENT OF MEDICALLY COMPLEX CHILDREN

ANN HOLMAN
PHYLLIS CHARLES
LEGERTHA BARNER

INTRODUCTION

A decent and compassionate society must ensure the safety and well-being of its children when their parents are not capable of doing so. In our society, this becomes the responsibility of the public child welfare system and social service providers (Harris, 1988). The mission of ensuring children's safety becomes increasingly difficult as one considers the growing numbers of medically complex children who require child welfare services. An increasing number of children with serious chronic illnesses are spending many months—in some cases their entire lives—in acute care hospitals because alternative home care is unavailable. Many of these children have complex medical conditions and/or health care needs often requiring high levels of techologic and nursing support. While these children have medical problems, they are alert, responsive and are first and foremost, children who would benefit from a nurturing family environment (Charles, Hochstadt & Yost, 1988).

Social service providers play a crucial role in the successful discharge, placement and support of these medically complex children in their birth families as well as in foster family homes. Discharge and follow-up of these youngsters require a coordinated effort on the part of medical personnel as well as hospital and child welfare social workers. Social workers need an understanding of the many medical as well as psychosocial needs of children and families. The authors of this chapter will address permanency planning for medically complex children, the recruitment and assessment of prospective foster/adoptive families, and discharge planning. The social worker's role in placing medically complex children is twofold; providing services to the child and family which will enhance the child's development and aiding families in accessing the many systems which impinge on them. To fulfill both these roles requires much time and dedication. However, it is well worth the effort to see once hospital-bound children thriving in a family environment.

Throughout this chapter, examples will be given from the authors' experiences in placing these special needs children and from the federally funded Medical Foster Parent Program (MFPP) of the Children's Home and Aid Society of Illinois and Aid Society of Illinois and La Rabida Children's Hospital and Research Center (Department of Health and Human Services, 1986).

PERMANENCY PLANNING

Permanency planning is perhaps best defined by Maluccio and Fein (1983) as, "a systematic process of carrying out, within a brief, time limited period, a set of goal directed activities designed to help children live in families that offer continuity of relationships with nurturing parents or caretakers and the opportunity to establish lifetime relationships." Public Law 96-272 (Social Security Act, 1935), is the benchmark legislation which provided the legislative framework for permanency planning. This law was passed just one year before Katie Beckett, the first home care ventilator-dependent child, was discharged from the hospital (Office of Technology Assessment, 1987). Thus, the thrust for permanency planning came at approximately the same time the financial and technological supports became available to provide home care for children with complex medical needs.

Public Law 96-272 (Social Security Act, 1935), contains a number of key components which directly impact social service providers and have special meaning for children with complex medical needs. Some of these provisions include:

• A case plan for each child describing the child's permanency goal and the proposed method of achieving permanency for the child.

• A six month review of the case plan to determine progress toward the stated permanency goal and progress made in correcting the conditions which led to a child's placement in substitute care.

- A judicial determination that reasonable efforts were made to prevent a child's out-of-home placement or to reunify the family once a child has been placed in substitute care.

- A dispositional hearing within eighteen months of a child's placement and periodically thereafter to determine the future status of the child.

- A provision for adoption assistance or subsidy to encourage the adoption of children who might not otherwise be adopted.

The first permanency goal in a case plan is generally "return home" (to the biological family). This goal is established upon a child's entrance into the child welfare system subsequent to an abuse or neglect report being filed. This goal of "return home" suggests that a child has already lived with his or her birth family. However, many of the medically complex children who were placed through the MFPP never lived outside the hospital with their families. The earliest part of their lives often was spent in intensive care nurseries. Thus, these children did not establish the normal bonding with their birth parents crucial to a child's subsequent development (Mahler, Pine & Bergman, 1975; Fraiberg, 1983). This lack of bonding also may inhibit a birth parent's attachment to his or her child and lessen a parent's motivation to visit their child on a regular basis, thus exacerbating the problem. By the time a child is medically stable and ready for discharge from the hospital, the birth parents may no longer be visiting a child on a regular basis and in some instances cannot be located.

Besides lack of bonding and attachment, a variety of factors serve to inhibit birth parents from visiting their medically complex children in the hospital: economic factors of getting to and from the hospital, difficulty finding child care for older children, substance abuse problems which inhibit their ability to function adequately, and guilt.

The hospital social worker should make reasonable efforts to enable the birth family to parent their child if at all possible. Such efforts may include: attempting to locate missing parents, establishing a training contract to teach parents the medical care of their child, making a determination as to whether a birth parent is capable of meeting a child's medical needs, and helping a parent access existing community resources which would enable them to care for their child at home. However, if such efforts fail to achieve reunification of a hospitalized child with his or her birth family, the child abuse and neglect hotline is called by the medical social worker and a medical neglect report is made. In Illinois, the Department of Children and Family Services

(DCFS) may then take custody of a child and a new focus on permanency planning begins—that of locating a foster family. The child then remains in the hospital or institution until an appropriate family resource can be located.

Since children wait in the hospital until a family can be found for them, it is critically important that specialized foster families are recruited to parent these medically complex youngsters. Not only can a family provide the essential one-on-one stimulation and attachment critical to a child's subsequent development, such a family resource also fulfills the mandates of Public Law 96-272 (Social Security Act, 1935), holding that a child should be placed in the least restrictive setting which most closely approximates a family. Other aspects of this law will be discussed later in the chapter.

RECRUITMENT AND ASSESSMENT OF FOSTER FAMILIES

Methods of Recruitment

One of the most integral roles of the social worker is that of recruitment of foster and adoptive families. When recruiting foster/adoptive families, social service personnel look for families that are currently a part of the established foster care system, go into the community to locate families that have previously fostered or adopted, or recruit families new to the child welfare system altogether.

In working with MFPP, it was found that successful recruitment needs to be child-specific. Families respond better to real, individualized children than to a general appeal to parent "medically complex youngsters." Thus, in any recruitment effort, it is vitally important for the social worker to be thoroughly acquainted with the child to successfully recruit a family. Acquainting oneself with a child may include: visiting the child in their hospital or institutional setting, obtaining a good photograph and, if possible, a videotape of the child, talking with persons providing services to the child (i.e., medical personnel, volunteers at the hospital, teachers), being clear as to the child's legal status and whether a child can be placed out of state, and knowing whether a child's medical condition will allow for placement with a single or two parent family. Once the social worker is able to get a sense of a child's personality and needs, they can use this knowledge to make that child "come alive" for families who are potential parents.

Initially social workers can contact former foster adoptive families who may be excellent resources not only as potential parents themselves, but also as recruiters for new families who may be able to parent these children. This is why it is imperative to maintain a good working rapport with these families. These parents can be "buddy families" to those who are just beginning the process by providing support and helping new families through rough times.

In addition to former foster adoptive families, child welfare social workers should also look to agencies that are known to have an adoption or foster care program which specialize in the recruitment of special needs children. It is very important that the agency have experience in working with these types of placements. This knowledge is needed in order to develop a program to assist families to meet the needs of medically complex children (Illinois Special Needs Adoption Project, 1987). The MFPP originally planned to recruit all the families from within one agency. However, it soon became apparent that it was necessary to utilize established foster families from other agencies to provide enough homes for these children.

Another ideal place to recruit families for these children is in the environment where the child is already known. Some families for medically complex children can be located within the pool of workers in a hospital or institutional setting. Hospital volunteers or health professionals who have become familiar with a child's medical care and develop a relationship with that child may be excellent candidates to provide foster care. In the MFPP five families were recruited for medically complex children in this manner. These people were familiar with the child's needs as well as the medical system. Thus, the medical aspect of a child's care did not seem as overwhelming or frightening for them. Even if these hospital personnel cannot, themselves, provide a home for a child, they can be an excellent source of recruitment for other families within their church or community. They often know the child best and can present the child as an individual rather than as a list of medical problems. It is also important that medical care providers who become foster parents are able to meet the child's emotional as well as physical needs. Children needing foster placements are dealing with issues of separation and loss and will need parents who can attend to these needs, and not merely the medical aspects of their care.

Jessica's foster family who had met her through their work at the hospital had no problems dealing with her bronchopulmonary dysplasia. However, they did have difficulty with Jessica's tantruming and could not set appropriate limits for her. Due to these problems, the foster family was referred for counseling services to learn effective behavioral modification techniques.

In addition to recruiting families from within the medical and foster care systems, the electronic and print media can be another effective means of recruitment. While radio and TV can reach large numbers of families, careful screening will need to follow such a media campaign to assess families' ability to meet the needs of medically complex children. For example, in the MFPP, twenty-eight families responded to an airing of a three-minute spot on the local TV news. However, none of these families actually went on to become specialized foster parents, although some were referred to regular foster care or adoption programs.

There were several reasons why families did not follow through to become specialized foster care provided in the above example. Single applicants may not have had the mandatory back-up caretaker to learn a child's tracheostomy or ventilator care. Other reasons given were related to issues of separation and loss. Some families could not consider becoming attached to a child only to have the child return to their biological family. Others could not consider the possibility, however remote, that the child could die while in their care.

Media efforts to recruit families for these children will be enhanced if the social worker can obtain a legal release to photograph the child in an attractive manner. Making children visible and educating prospective parents to the joys and challenges of parenting medically complex children can be helpful. While the MFPP did not find large media efforts to be immediately successful in locating appropriate families for children, these larger scale efforts may be effective in the long run. Families often may hear an ad and consider fostering or adopting for months or even years before they actually take the step to contact an agency.

Recruitment in local newspapers or in targeted periodicals such as nursing journals can also be an effective means of finding homes for these youngsters. Local newspaper columns such as "Tuesday's Child" which help highlight specific children needing homes have also proved effective if they have an appealing description and picture of a child. These efforts often elicit calls from potential families, not only for that child, but for other children who may have similar problems.

Featuring children in local and national adoption exchanges (if a child is legally free for adoption or able to be listed) can be yet another effective means of recruitment for these children. Even if the birth parents' rights have not been terminated, and thus children are not legally free for adoption, children may be able to be featured in newsletters of various associations such as the Council on Adoptable Children (COAC) if the children's legal status is made clear. Other newsletters, such as those of the United Cerebral Palsy Association, may be the recruitment mode of choice depending on the child's specific medical problems.

To ignore the changing face of the American family is to ignore potential familial resources for children who need homes. Since the fabric of our society is changing, the "family" is no longer exclusively defined as a mother, a father and the children. It is well a known fact that many of the households in America are now headed by a single parent, usually a female. Thus, many agencies have reviewed their policies and practices, such as restrictive income or age requirements, which in the past have screened out appropriate families for children. Now less importance is placed on a family's home and financial or marital status and more attention is paid to a family's stability and ability to meet a child's needs.

Assessment of Prospective Foster Families

After recruiting potential families, the social worker conducts a comprehensive assessment of the parents. The child is then matched with a family who can best meet his or her unique medical and psychosocial needs. A typical family assessment should include (Children's Home and Aid Society of Illinois, 1987):

- Current family composition
- Description of the home and neighborhood
- Parent's background history
- Current marriage and/or history of family life
- Attitudes and capacities
- Social worker's evaluation

While there are many qualities which are necessary for families who are considering substitute parenting, there are several which have been found to be especially important in foster families who successfully parent medically complex children. One quality social workers should look for is the ability of the parents to organize their lives and deal with a large number of systems. A family of a medically complex youngster may need to interface with nursing agencies, equipment companies, numerous health care professionals, the Division of Services for Crippled Children (or comparable state agency), and the child welfare system (this, in itself, includes social workers, the juvenile court, and the child's birth parents). Foster families need somewhat structured and organized lives to successfully deal with all these systems. Openness and flexibility on the part of the child and family is required.

Other qualities which are helpful for these families to possess include patience, a sense of humor, a desire and ability to nurture, and empathy for the child and his or her birth family. Being able to deal with crises and having sufficient physical stamina to meet the needs of a particular child are also important qualities. Foster parents need to possess the ability to work with birth parents, the ability to "let go" if a child is to return home, or the ability to form lasting relationships if they proceed to adopt the child. (Illinois Special Needs Adoption Project, 1987).

Families wanting to parent medically complex children have a variety of motives for doing so. Most often, foster parents are well intentioned; wanting to help the most helpless in our society. Other motives may include: restoring the equilibrium in a marital relationship, the gratification received from parenting a dependent child, or a change in the family's life style. For example, one single foster parent applicant wanted to parent a medically complex child when her own daughter left home for college. Some families want to parent medically complex youngers as a means of "giving back" to society. Whether that need is based in a religious value or out of a sense of guilt, many families feel the need to do something useful for the community (Burke & Dawson, 1987).

Whatever their motivations, families providing foster care for medically complex children are risk takers. They are parenting children who may not get better and indeed in some cases may die while in their care. Therefore, it is essential that these families have a good support system to help them with both their emotional and physical needs.

DISCHARGE PLANNING

While a child welfare social worker is doing the assessment of a potential family in the community, the medical social worker is working with the health care system to effect the child's discharge from the hospital.

The primary role of the medical social worker is that of case management: helping the family access the medical system, referring to, and coordinating with, the many agencies needed in the placement of the medically complex child, and aiding in the provision of psychosocial support and counseling.

Foremost, the family needs to feel comfortable within the medical system, which can be complex and sometimes intimidating. An introduction to the child's health care providers by the social worker is essential. The social worker should set up an initial meeting with these primary professionals as soon as possible. The prospective family can then acquaint themselves with the team (e.g., physicians, rehabilitation specialists, nurse discharge planner) and begin to become a working member of it.

During this meeting, the child's medical/developmental history and current needs should be discussed and outlined. Parents will need to have this reviewed and updated a number of times during the discharge process and will require a basic understanding of these conditions. Next, the social worker, along with the health care personnel, needs to help the family accept and understand the physical condition of the child. While some of the children who have tracheostomies may be decannulated and lead relatively normal lives, the condition of other children needing placement may not improve or may deteriorate. Allowing the family to see the child and his/her medical equipment will help the family better understand the child's medical needs. Another goal of the initial meeting is to set up the parent's training schedule so they can learn to care for the child's medical, rehabilitation and psychological needs. The social worker, a discharge planner and/or primary nurse from the hospital, can set up these sessions. The length of training will vary depending on the child's needs and the family's learning style. During the training process, the social worker will need to identify and clarify roles with the staff and the foster family. The staff and the foster family will need to work closely together and thus a clear definition of roles is necessary. Often times, when a child has been hospitalized for a considerable length of time, the hospital staff may feel as if they are the child's family, especially if the birth family has not visited the child on a regular basis. The adoptive or foster family may be seen as intruding on this relationship. If this occurs, both the staff and family will need help in resolving this issue and in defining appropriate roles. Staff may need to ventilate their feelings of loss and separation while families will need to see why the hospital staff may seem to be judging them or sometimes even alienating them. Helping the health care team to see discharge and placement of medically complex children as positive and helping them to resolve their own feelings of loss, is a necessary task for the medical social worker.

Medical and child welfare social workers also need to assist the families of medically complex youngsters to access educational, financial and health care resources. Childen with medically complex needs may require special educational help. Under the Public Law 94-142, (Education of the Handicapped Act, 1970) and Public Law 99-457 (Education of the Handicapped Act, 1970), children from zero to twenty-one years of age are guaranteed a free and appropriate education. However, it is not uncommon for conflicts to arise and for delays to be experienced in accessing these educational services for children.

> Bobby, a seven-year-old with bronchopulmonary dysplasia (BPD), subglottic stenosis and a tracheostomy was hospitalized for over three years waiting for a family. At the age of four, while still in the hospital, Bobby attended a school for the physically handicapped. He eventually was placed in a suburban foster/adoptive home. Due to the suburban school district's reluctance to allocate funds for a physically handicapped child with his needs, it took over a year to access an appropriate educational program for Bobby.

Medically complex children may be eligible for special education services if they have deficits in vision, hearing, behavior, health/physical impairments, speech, cognition, or learning. An Individualized Education Plan (IEP) is required to be written to meet a child's educational needs. This plan should be developed and reviewed annually. Parents will need to be assertive and knowledgeable about these provisions and may require the assistance of the social worker in setting up meetings with school personnel and preparing for an IEP. Local parent coalition groups such as Chicago's Coordinating Council for Handicapped Children can assist in this area. The Coordinating Council provides information to parents on educational rights as well as advocacy services and parent/professional training workshops (a list of parent training centers is included in Appendix A).

There are many financial concerns that may confront the family of the medically complex child. One, certainly, is the cost of health care. In Illinois, the Department of Public Aid along with the Division of

Services for Crippled Children (DSCC) can offer continuous nursing services which not only provides medical support for the family, but can also relieve the stress that sometimes accompanies caring for a child with medical problems. Since most insurances will not cover pre-existing conditions, this service is much needed. Once again, every state does not provide the same services and the social worker will need to help the family to obtain services that may be available in their areas.

Supplemental Security Income (SSI) is another financial resource that may be available to the medically complex child. This program, administered through the Social Security Administration, provides additional income to qualifying handicapped individuals and is dependent on the child's medical condition and family income. The social worker should refer families to this agency if they meet the eligibility requirements. Another source of financial support, an adoption assistance or adoption subsidy, will be discussed later in this chapter.

Since the medically complex child will need specialized health care, helping the family find appropriate care is paramount. Many times the family will continue to be followed by the discharging hospital. This, of course, is the simplest option since the medical staff will be familiar with the child and the family and the family will be familiar with the facility. If the family chooses to be followed elsewhere, good coordination and follow-up is essential. Medical records, developmental history, and rehabilitation needs should be communicated to the new physician and other specialists. The social worker, along with the discharge planner and physician, should coordinate this transfer. In some states a state agency such as Services for Crippled Children may also help with this transition and follow-up through their case management services. Respite care should also be investigated prior to the discharge so the foster family will have this service available to them when needed.

Not only are the needs of the child important, but the psychosocial needs of the family need to be addressed. To provide ongoing support for the family, networking with other families who have been through the same process is recommended. The social worker should link up new families with experienced families that are known to the facility, or refer the family to a more formal network through an established support group such as SKIP (Sick Kids Need Involved People). This group, started in Washington, D.C., is now nationally known and has chapters throughout the country. In either instance, families can find support and identify with those who have "been there." Problems such as physical adaptations of the home environment and lifestyle changes can be shared and possible solutions found.

Racial issues may be encountered when working with hard to place children. In some communities, minority children are over represented in this population. This provides a challenge to child welfare personnel to locate families of racial and ethnic compatibility. Despite the best efforts transracial placements may have to be considered. There are unique issues that can arise in this type of placement. Social workers need to be aware of racial differences and should be culturally competent in their work with families.

Counseling is another psychosocial service that the social worker can provide for the child and family. A child may be experiencing feelings of abandonment, low self-esteem, or apprehension about a new placement. Families may need help dealing with the child's emotional or behavioral problems as well as the stress of caring for a medically complex child. For these reasons, counseling should be offered to those who require it. If not accepted initially, it may be offered again at various times during the placement process, when stressors may be higher and the family more receptive.

ALTERNATIVE CARE

Once a family has been trained in a particular child's care and the child is discharged into the family's home, permanency planning becomes an ongoing process.

After a child is in the foster care system, the two most common permanency goals are: return home and adoption. The first permanency goal is almost always return home to the birth family. To facilitate this goal, the child welfare social worker meets with the birth parents to establish a case plan. This plan, which is one of the components of Public Law 96-272 (Social Security Act, 1935) outlines several objectives for a parent to help them achieve reunification. Several specific tasks are then outlined under each objective. For example, one objective may be for a parent to develop and maintain a relationship with their child through regular visitation. The tasks may include visiting a child on a weekly basis.

If, over a reasonable period of time, a family is not able to make use of the reunification services provided or if the goal of reunification is no longer appropriate, the permanency goal may then be changed to adoption at an administrative case review which is held every six months for each child. This review was also established as a result of Public Law 96-272 (Social Security Act, 1935). In Illinois, a child's foster family is given the first option to adopt a child if he or she has been in the home for at least a year. Every attempt is made to provide a long-term, consistent legal status for a child. This helps to maintain as much continuity and stability as possible in the lives of foster children and their families.

Moves from hospitals to foster homes and changes in legal status can be very confusing for a child. One of the ways social workers can help a child make sense of the many moves he or she may have made is by compiling a life book for the child. A life book details a child's history and prepares him/her to move into a foster or adoptive home. A medically complex child's life book may include various medical facilities in which a child may have lived. A life book also explains in simple language the reason why a child is being adopted and what adoption means.

There are several ways that a child may be freed for adoption. First, a child can be freed through the voluntary surrender of parental rights on the part of one or both of the birth parents. If only one parent surrenders, the social worker makes an all out effort to locate the other parent to assess their interest in parenting or surrendering their child.

The second method of freeing a child for adoption is through the termination of parental rights. Preparing a case for termination includes documenting all efforts that were made to provide services to a birth family and illustrating that, based on a stated termination of parental rights statute, there is enough evidence to do so. While statutory grounds for termination vary from state to state, common grounds may include failure to maintain a reasonable degree of interest in a child or failure to correct the conditions which led to a child's placement. Once parental rights have been terminated, a child is legally free and is available for adoption by his or her foster family.

Most adoptive families who undertake the care of a medically complex child cannot afford the full expense of that child's care. Families' private insurance rarely provides coverage for preexisting conditions and the state's Medicaid program may not cover the full cost of necessary adjunct services such as speech or physical therapy and counseling. Therefore, in all states adoption assistance or subsidy is available based on the child's unique needs. This assistance is mandated through Public Law 96-272 (Social Security Act, 1935) to encourage the adoption of children who might not otherwise be adopted and is reassessed annually.

CONCLUSION

As has been demonstrated, the role of the social service provider is multifaceted. To adequately assist families in the parenting of medically complex youngsters, social workers must have a working knowledge of the medical, education, financial and child welfare systems. They also need to be sensitive to the changing physical and emotional needs of these children and their families. Children will thrive in an environment where their parents have a healthy self-esteem and a belief in their ability to manage (Weissbourd, 1988). If families are adequately supported, this can lead to an expansion of the number of families who opt to care for medically complex children in their homes and in so doing facilitate more successful placements of these children (Massachusetts Department of Public Health, 1987).

REFERENCES

Burke, M., & Dawson, T. A. (1987). Temporary care foster parents: Motives and issues of separation and loss. *Child and Adolescent Social Work, 4*, 30–38.

Charles, P., Hochstadt, N. J., & Yost, D. M. (1988). Medical foster care: Achieving permanency for seriously ill children. *Children Today, 17* (5), 22–26.

Children's Home and Aid Society of Illinous (1987). *Guide to the Content of a Home Study*. Unpublished Manuscript. Chicago, IL.

Department of Health and Human Services (1986). *Medical foster care for seriously chronically medically ill children*. (Grant No. 90-CW-0790). Washington, DC: Office of Human Development Services, Administration for Children Youth and Families.

Fraiberg, S. H. (1959). *The Magic Years*. New York: Charles Scriber's Sons.

Harris, D. V. (1988). Renewing our commitment of child welfare. *Social Work, 33*, (6), 483–484.

Illinois Special Needs Adoption Project (1977). *Possible recruitment approaches to potential foster and adoptive families for children with developmental disabilities, medical complex conditions and chronic illness*. Unpublished Manuscript. Chicago, IL.

Mahler, M. S., Pine, F., & Bergman, A. (1975). *The Psychological Birth of the Human Infant*. New York: Basic Books.

Maluccio, A. N., & Fein, E. L. (1983). Permanency planning: a redefinition. *Child Welfare, 62* (3), 195–201.

Massachusetts Department of Public Health (June 9, 1987). *Child Welfare grantees meeting notes*, Washington, D.C.

Office of Technology Assessment (1987). *Technology dependent children: Hospital, home care—a technical memorandum* (Office of Technology Assessment, U.S. Congress, No. OTA-TM-H-38). Washington, D.C.: U.S. Government Printing Office.

Social Security Act of 1935, 602 U.S.C.§402 Title IV (1980).

The Education of the Handicapped Act of 1970, 20 U.S.C.§1400 (1975).

Weissbourd, B., & Patrick, M. (1988). In the best interest of the family: The emergence of family resource programs. *Infants and Young Children, 1* (2), 46–54.

APPENDIX A. PARENT COALITION GROUPS

ALABAMA

Special Educational Action Committee, Inc.
2970 Cottage Hill Road
Suite 163
Mobile, Alabama 36606
(205) 478-1208
(800) 222-7322

ALASKA

Southeast Regional Resource Center
210 Ferry Way, Suite 200
Juneau, Alaska 99801
(907) 586-6806

ARIZONA

Pilot Parents, Inc.
2005 North Central #100
Phoenix, Arizona 85004
(602) 271-4012

ARKANSAS

Focus Inc.
2917 King Street, Suite C
Jonesboro, Arkansas 72401
(501) 935-2750

Arkansas Coalition for the Handicapped
519 East Fifth Street
Little Rock, Arkansas 72402
(501) 376-0378

CALIFORNIA

Multicultural Impact, Inc.
University Affiliated Program
Children's Hospital of L.A.
Post Office Box 54700
Los Angeles, California 90054
(213) 669-2300

Parents Helping Parents
535 Race St. #220
San Jose, Calif. 95126
(408) 288-5010

Project COPE
9160 Monte Vista Ave.
Montclair, Calif. 91763
(714) 985-3116

Teams of Advocates for Special Kids (TASK)
18685 Santa Ynez
Fountain Valley, Calif. 92708
(714) 962-6332

COLORADO

Denver Association for Retarded Citizens
899 Logan
Suite 311
Denver, Colorado 80203
(303) 831-7733

Parent Education and Assistance for Kids
6055 Lehman Drive #101
Colorado Springs, Colorado 80918
(719) 531-9400

CONNECTICUT

Connecticut Parent Advocacy Center
Post Office Box 579
East Lyme, Connecticut 06333
(203) 886-5250
(800) 445-2722

DELAWARE

Parent Information Center of Delaware
325 East Main Street
Suite 203
Newark, Delaware 19711
(302) 366-0152

DISTRICT OF COLUMBIA

Parents Reaching Out Service
DC General Hospital
Department of Pediatrics
4th Floor, West Wing
1900 Massachusetts Avenue, S.E.
Washington, D.C. 20003
(202) 546-8847

FLORIDA

Broader Opportunities for the Learning Disabled (B.O.L.D.)
Post Office Box 546309
Surfside, Florida 33154
(305) 866-3262

Parent Education Network/Florida
2215 East Henry Avenue
Tampa, Florida 33610
(813) 239-1179

GEORGIA

Parents Educating Parents (PEP)
Association for Retarded Citizens of Georgia
1851 Ram Runway
College Park, Georgia 30337
(404) 761-2745
Specialized Training of Military Parents (East)
1851 Ram Runway
College Park, Georgia 30337
(404) 767-2258

ILLINOIS

Coordinating Council for Handicapped Children
20 East Jackson, Room 900
Chicago, Illinois 60604
(312) 939-3513 (Voice)
(312) 939-3519 (TDD)

Designs for Change
220 South State Street
Suite 1900
Chicago, Illinois 60604
(312) 922-0317

Keshet
Jewish Parents of Children with Special Needs
Post Office Box 59065
Chicago, Illinois 60645
(312) 588-0551

Parentele
8331 Kimball Avenue
Skokie, Illinois 60076
(312) 677-3796

Parents of Chronically Ill Children
29 Lovell Valley Drive
Springfield, Illinois 62702
(217) 522-6810

INDIANA

Task Force on Education for the Handicapped, Inc.
833 Northside Boulevard
Building #1 Rear
South Bend, Indiana 46617-2993
(219) 234-7101

IOWA

Iowa Pilot Parents
33 North 12th Street
Post Office Box 1151
Fort Dodge, Iowa 50501
(515) 576-5870
Pilot Parents
1000 Sims
Council Bluffs, Iowa 51501
(712) 621-3884

KANSAS

Families Together, Inc.
Box 86153
Topeka, Kansas 66686
(913) 273-6343

KENTUCKY

Kentucky Coalition for Career and Leisure Development
366 Waller Avenue
Suite 119
Lexington, Kentucky 40504
(606) 278-4712

MAINE

Maine Parent Federation, Inc.
Post Office Box 2067
Augusta, Maine 04330
(207) 582-2504
(800) 325-0220

SPIN (Special-Needs Parent Information Network)
Post Office Box 2067
Augusta, Maine 04330
(207) 582-2504
(800) 325-0220

MASSACHUSETTS

Federation for Children with Special Needs
312 Stuart Street Second Floor
Boston, Massachusetts 02116
(617) 482-2915

Technical Assistance for Parent Programs (TAPP)
312 Stuart Street Second Floor
Boston, Massachusetts 02116
(617) 482-2915

MICHIGAN

Citizens Alliance to Uphold Special Education (CAUSE)
Parents Training Program
313 South Washington Street
Suite 400
Lansing, Michigan 48933
(517) 485-4084

United Cerebral Palsy Association/ Detroit Community Service Department
17000 West Eight Mile Road
Suite 380
Southfield, Michigan 48075
(313) 557-5070

MINNESOTA

Parent Advocacy Coalition for Educational Rights
Pacer Center, Inc.
4826 Chicago Avenue
Minneapolis, Minnesota 55417
(612) 827-2966

MISSISSIPPI

Association of Developmental Organizations of Mississippi
6055 Highway 18S
Suite A
Jackson, Mississippi 39209
(601) 922-3210

Mississippi Parent Advocacy Center
6055 Highway 18 S.
Jackson, Mississippi 39209
(601) 922-3210

Parents, Let's Unite for Kids
1500 North 30th Street
Billings, Montana 59101
(406) 657-2055

Involve New Jersey, Inc.
26 C2 East 2nd Street
Moorestown, New Jersey 08057
(609) 778-0599

New Hampshire Coalition for Handicapped Citizens, Inc.
Parent Information Center
Post Office Box 1422
Concord, New Hampshire 03302
(603) 224-7005

Technical Assistance to Parent Programs Project (T.A.P.P.P.)
Post Office Box 1422
Concord, New Hampshire 03302
(603) 224-6299

Protection and Advocacy System
2201 San Pedro N.E.
Building 4, #140
Albuquerque, New Mexico 87110
(505) 888-0111

Southwest Communication Resources, Inc.
Post Office Box 788
Bernalillo, New Mexico 87004
(505) 867-3396

Parent's Information Group for Exceptional Children, Inc.
129 Cheerwood Drive
Baldwinsville, New York 13027
(315) 423-2735

Parents Coalition for Education of New York City
24-16 Bridge Plaza South
Lobby Floor
Long Island, New York 11101
(718) 729-8866

Parent Network Center
1443 Main Street
Buffalo, New York 14209
(716) 885-1004

Parents of Galactosemic Children, Inc.
1 Ash Court
New City, New York 10056

Western New York Association for the Learning Disabled
255 Elmwood Street
Kenmore, New York 14217
(716) 874-7200

Nevada Association for the Handicapped
6200 West Oakey Boulevard
Las Vegas, Nevada 89102-1142
(702) 870-7050

Advocacy Center for Children's Education and Parent Training (A.C.C.E.P.T.)
Post Office Box 10565
Raleigh, North Carolina 27605
(919) 294-5266

Exceptional Children's Advocacy Council
Post Office Box 16
Davidson, North Carolina 28036
(704) 892-1321

Parents Project
300 Enola Road
Morganton, North Carolina 28655
(704) 433-2864

OHIO

National Parent CHAIN, Inc.
933 High Street
Suite 106
Worthington, Ohio 43805
(614) 431-1307 (Voice and TDD)
**Ohio Coalition for the Education
of Handicapped Children**
933 High Street
Suite 106
Worthington, Ohio 43805
(614) 431-1307

Support Group for Monosomy 9P
c/o Jonathan Storr
43304 Kipton Nickle Plate Road
LaGrange, Ohio 44050
(216) 775-4255

**Tri-state Organized Coalition for
Persons with Disabilities**
SOC Information Center
3333 Vine Street
Suite 604
Cincinnati, Ohio 45220
(513) 861-2400

OREGON

**Coalition in Oregon for Parent
Education (COPE)**
999 Locust Street, N.E., #42
Salem, Oregon 97303
(503) 373-7477 (Voice/TDD)

PENNSYLVANIA

**Association for Retarded Citizens/
Allegheny**
1001 Brighton Road
Pittsburgh, Pennsylvania 15233
(412) 322-6008

**PA Association for Children and
Adults with Learning Disabilities**
Box 208
Uwchland, Pennsylvania 19408
(215) 458-8193

Parent Education Network
240 Haymeadow Drive
York, Pennsylvania 17402
(717) 845-9722
(800) 522-5827

Parents Union for Public Schools
401 North Broad Street, Room
916
Philadelphia, Pennsylvania 19108
(215) 574-0337

PUERTO RICO

**Asociacion de Padres Pro Beinstar
d Ninos Impedidos de Puerto Rico,
Inc. (APNI)**
Box 21301
Rio Piedras, P.R. 00928
(809) 765-0345
(809) 763-4665

SOUTH DAKOTA

South Dakota Parent Connection
Post Office Box 84813
Sioux Falls, S.D. 57118-4813

TENNESSEE

E.A.C.H., Inc.
Post Office Box 121257
Nashville, Tennessee 37212
(615) 298-1080
(800) 342-1660 (Voice/TTY)

TEXAS

Advocacy, Inc.
7800 Shoal Creek Boulevard,
171E
Austin, Texas 78757
(512) 454-4816

Association for Retarded Citizens of Texas, Inc.
833 Houston Street
Austin, Texas 78756
(512) 454-6694

Early Parent Intervention Association for Retarded Citizens of Texas
910 Seventh Street
Orange, Texas 77630
(409) 886-1363

Path
6465 Calder Avenue
Suite 202
Beaumont, Texas 77707
(409) 866-4726

UTAH

Utah Parent Information & Training Center
4984 South 300 W
Murray, Utah 84107
(801) 265-9883
(800) 468-1160

Parents Involved in Education Developmental Center for Handicapped Persons
Utah State University
DCHP UMC 6580
Logan, Utah 84322
(801) 750-1172

VERMONT

Vermont Association for Retarded Citizens
37 Champlain Mill
Winooski, Vermont 05404
(802) 655-4016

VIRGINIA

Parent Education Advocacy Training Center
228 South Pitt Street
Suite 300
Alexandria, Virignia 22314
(203) 836-2953

WASHINGTON

Parent to Parent Support ARC of King County
2230 Eighth Avenue
Seattle, Washington 98121
(206) 461-7800

Specialized Training of Military Parents (West)
12208 Pacific Highway, S.W.
Tacoma, Washington 98499
(206) 588-1741

Washington PAVE Parent-to-Parent Training Project
6316 South 12th
Tacoma, Washington 98465
(206) 565-2266 (Voice/TDD)

WISCONSIN

Parent Education Project United Cerebral Palsy of Southeastern Wisconsin
230 West Wells Street, #502
Milwaukee, Wisconsin 53203
(414) 272-4500/1077 (TTY)
(800) 472-5525

CHAPTER 7

ACCESSING THE EDUCATION SYSTEM FOR STUDENTS WHO REQUIRE HEALTH TECHNOLOGY AND TREATMENT

TERRY HEINTZ CALDWELL
KATHRYN A. KIRKHART

INTRODUCTION

Children who require health technology and treatment have special needs. The population of children requiring health technology and treatment has been defined by the Office of Technology Assessment (1987) and also the Task Force on Technology-Dependent Children (1988) as persons with chronic disabilities requiring routine use of a particular medical device to compensate for the loss of a life sustaining body function and who require daily ongoing care or monitoring by trained personnel. For these children to live fully integrated lives within a family and community context, the educational system must serve students in least-restrictive settings. Therefore, the education system with providers of care and family members must work together to support an intricate group of services designed to meet the educational needs of each child.

There is no single model of care for providing services to children who require health technology and treatment. Various models have evolved within communities depending upon resources and needs (Aday, Aitken, & Wegener, 1988). For children cared for at home, a family-centered system of care is emerging (Shelton, Jeppson, & Johnson, 1987). Families are central in decision-making, managing, and providing care. They provide informed consent during hospital discharge planning and educational planning efforts. The family weighs the risks and benefits of various procedures and determines the acceptability of each for their own child.

Foster families usually have less personal decision-making power and must work within the foster care system and with designated authorities to understand and deal with finer points of medical risk and benefit. Hochstadt & Yost (1989) outline general foster care issues for medically complex children. A Louisiana student in foster care who uses a ventilator to breathe has a team of individuals involved in decision-making for her ongoing educational services. The team includes a judge, a state social worker, foster parents, a surrogate parent, a legal advocate, a physician, a nurse case manager, special education coordinator, and others.

This chapter presents issues involved in the provision of educational services for students who require health technology assistance and treatment, including those who are in foster care. The Louisiana model of services (Kirkhart, Steele, Pomeroy, Anguzza, French, & Gates, 1988; Kirkhart & Gates, 1988) is used as a reference while other national models are also noted.

EDUCATION AND THE LAW

Many children who use health technology and treatment do not have access to an education which is similar to the education provided to their peers. Prior to 1976, this had been true for children with a variety of special needs who received limited education in settings which were often isolated. The passage of PL 94-142, The Education of All Handicapped Act (1975) provided the opportunity for handicapped children to participate in school programs. The law, which mandated education in the least restrictive environment, opened the doors of schools to children with a variety of handicapping conditions, including those with severe impairments.

School programs for children with special health needs are addressed in PL 94-142. These students are provided access to special education services if they qualify as "Other Health Impaired." The classification of "Other Health Impaired" is based on a student's reduced vitality, physiological limitations and overall inability to appropriately access educational services to benefit from education. Despite the "Other Health Impaired" classification, children with special health needs, especially those who require health technology or procedures, have not been consistently provided the opportunity to receive special education services in the least restrictive environment (LRE).

A 1985 study demonstrates that most states are not administratively prepared to manage children with special health conditions. The survey shows that 13 states have no written guidelines for administration of health procedures in school, 18 have miscellaneous guidelines, and only 6 have complete guidelines. "Despite progressive state and federal legislation during the past decade, mandating equal education for all children, in particular PL 94-142, there remains serious questions about implementation of these laws with regard to medically involved children" (Wood, Walker, & Gardner, 1986, p. 215).

Lawsuits relating to school attendance with appropriate services have been noted by Sokoloff, Lewis, Lynch, & Murphy (1986) and Vitello (1987). Most suits have been brought against school districts using arguments based on PL 94-142 or Section 504 federal requirements as they relate to special education or access to regular education. Case law has not yet established standard practices for the education of these children. It has, however, clarified some basic points. In Irving Independent School District v. Tatro (1984), it has been determined that clean intermittent catheterization is a "related service" that must be provided under PL 94-142 (Vitello, 1987). In Elizabeth S. v. Gilhool (1987), it has been established that services must be provided to children with health or physical impairments who do not require special education (Sokoloff, Lewis, Lynch, & Murphy, 1986). The decision of Detsel v. Board of Education of the Auburn Enlarged City School District (1986, 1987) has deemed that constant care by a LPN/RN is "medical" and need not be provided by the school under PL 94-142. In Macomb County Intermediate School District v. Joshua S. the court disagreed with the decision in Detsel stating that the court had failed to adhere to a principle developed in Tatro. Tatro established that services are "medical" only if they require provision by a licensed physician (Reiser, 1989).

Some states and/or individual school systems are successfully developing school programs. These systems blend resources and provide safe care in unique ways. For example, Louisiana's State Department of Education and the local school system blend funds to pay the salaries of caregivers; training of caregivers and other education staff is provided by a Title XIX funded case management program for ventilator-users. Illinois' educators pay for teachers' salaries while Public Assistance pays for the salaries of nurses who provide direct care in school. Policies for implementing LRE are evolving. For some

Table 7.1. Medically Fragile Students: Educational Issues.

1. Determining eligibility for special education services
2. Providing related and non-educational services
3. Assuring equal access to appropriate educational settings in the least restrictive environment
4. Promoting a safe learning environment
5. Assuring that health care services are delivered by appropriate and adequately trained personnel
6. Establishing support systems for staff, students, and families
7. Including appropriate information about students with specialized health care needs in inservice, preservice, and continuing education programs
8. Providing appropriate and safe transporation
9. Promoting research that assesses current and future delivery models

Note. From *The Report of the Council for Exceptional Children's Ad Hoc Committee on Medically Fragile Students* (p. 2–6) CEC. by the Council for Exceptional Children, 1988, Reston, Virginia: Reprinted by permission.

students LRE is interpreted as met when a student is in a hospital-based program, a home program, or a special education school. However, for most students LRE is usually met only when special resources are used for the student to attend regular classes in neighborhood schools; this setting is the *least* restrictive.

EDUCATIONAL ISSUES

Educational programs in the least restrictive environment are not a reality for many technology assisted children. In recognition of the serious nature of the issues, the Council for Exceptional Children (CEC) has convened a team of educational experts. This task force has examined issues which hinder implementation of LRE for children with special health conditions (Sirvos, 1988). These issues are listed in Table 7.1.

EDUCATIONAL PLANNING

In the State of Louisiana every school age child who is ventilated and medically stable attends school and participates in a relevant education program. Most students over the age of five years are in regular classrooms. As in most states, major issues and barriers emerge regarding provision of educational services. The action steps as identified by Louisiana State and Local Education agencies and health personnel are described below.

(1) Philosophy of Care: The Louisiana State Department of Education (SEA) assists the state's local school system in the implementation of LRE. SEA officials work with personnel of the statewide pediatric Ventilator Assisted Care Program to determine which school options are available and safe for children who use ventilators. As a result, the SEA has developed a policy endorsing placement in an educationally relevant program with access to resources to manage health care.

(2) Orientation of Health and Educational Personnel: Many health care providers who work with children using ventilators are accustomed to dealing with these children in intensive care or acute care hospital settings. As a result, they are uncomfortable with home care and community-based settings. In addition, they are often unfamiliar with the acquired abilities of schools to provide services and fear for the "safety" of the child in school. Louisiana tertiary care physicians and health care providers specializing in care of children who use technology meet with community-based physicians and health care personnel to provide information about safe school programs for these children (Caldwell, Todaro, & Gates, 1989). Educational personnel have been equally resistant since many have no experience administering school programs for children who use health technology. Historically, school systems have not been equipped to provide a safe environment for these children. Many school personnel do not know what support they need from health personnel or what other resources they need to implement programs. In recognition of these problems, the Louisiana Ventilator Assisted Care Program and Chronic Illness Program provide orientation for education personnel. Orientation includes information regarding the needs of the population, successful strategies for school involvement, assurances of support from families and health providers, and linkages with other school personnel who have experience in providing education services (Caldwell, Todaro, & Gates, 1990).

(3) Family Orientation and Support: Some families do not support or advocate for education in the least restrictive environment. Family members can be ambivalent because of their own fears as well as fears of health and education personnel who advise them. Students who use health technology have usually experienced at least one serious health crisis. It has been difficult for some families to move from the uncertain prognosis in intensive care to the bustling school setting.

Table 7.2. Students With Health-Impairments at School.
Reducing the Risk of Liability in the Classroom.

1. Obtain individualized prescriptions and protocols for procedures to be performed.
2. Review protocols approved by the physician with parents and have them sign form indicating their agreement with the procedures outlined in the protocol.
3. Document that appropriate training based on protocols has occurred. Include persons' names, specific procedures demonstrated, and date of scheduled rechecks.
4. Train anyone who will be involved in the child's care, i.e. bus driver, etc.
5. Establish contingency plans. Train other personnel who will take over when the major caregivers are not available and who will be available to assist major caregiver in an emergency situation.
6. Include maintenance and emergency procedures in your training.
7. Develop plans with physicians and parents for transport and provision of service in local emergency room.
8. Provide information to agencies providing services to the school (i.e. electric and telephone companies) to advise them of the need for priority service restorations.
9. Provide information to agencies interacting with the school during natural disasters (i.e. Fire Department, Red Cross) to acquaint them with the student's participation in a particular school and the needs that student will have during an emergency.
10. Effectively document needs and how they will be met in the IEP (Individual Education Plan).

Note: From *The Community Provider's Guide: An Information Outline for Working with Children with Special Needs in the Community* (p. V 2) by T. Caldwell, A. Todaro, and A.J. Gates, 1989, New Orleans, Louisiana: Children's Hospital. Reprinted by permission.

(4) School System Liability: Liability for the care of children who use health technology or procedures is the number one deterrent to education in the LRE. In Louisiana, guidelines to assist in assuring safe settings while reducing the probability of negligence have been devised; attorneys affiliated with the SEA assisted in the development. These are listed in Table 7.2. These guidelines reassure school personnel and set standards for care.

(5) Model for Decision-Making Regarding Appropriateness of School Participation: Should every child using health technology be in school? What are the major factors in decision-making? There have not been adequate parameters to use in decision-making regarding the appropriateness of school participation. In Louisiana, guidelines now recommend these decisions be made by a team comprised of family, health, education, and other personnel. When the child is in foster care, a surrogate parent is often involved. Some states require surrogate parents to be involved in educational planning when a student is a ward of the state (Louisiana's Law for Exceptional Students, 1983). In addition, the court or other foster care authorities have opinions regarding

school participation. The team evaluates the safety of providing school services on the basis of the stability of the child. It should be noted that participation decisions are *not* based on the student's cognitive function; placement issues are addressed later in this chapter.

(6) Systems of Collaboration which Address Program and Fiscal Responsibility: Financial support may not be readily available to implement the selected school program. There is no national consensus among policy-makers as to fiscal responsibility for the provision of personnel to provide health maintenance procedures at school. Successful models in various states or school districts have been creative in developing fiscal resources. Most use some interagency collaboration. Some states combine federal, state, and local education funds. Medicaid, Title V Children's Medical Services Program, or private sector funds may be involved.

(7) Classroom Resource Needs: An immediate problem in the inability of the teacher to "teach" if health maintenance procedures take up too much of the teacher's time. Louisiana LEA's and SEA's review requests for extra classroom personnel on a case by case basis. Personnel decisions are based on the amount of care a student requires, the number of personnel already in the classroom, and the emergency reaction time needed. For example, if a student has a tracheostomy, coughs up mucus secretions without needing suctioning, and can be without the tracheostomy for long periods of time, extra personnel are usually not recommended. If a student requires catheterization and is in a class with a classroom assistant who could assist in the completion of that catheterization, then extra personnel are not usually recommended. If a student is ventilator assisted, has a tracheostomy, and requires suctioning, ventilator checks, positioning, pressure relief, gastrostomy feeding, assistance with any academic or self-help endeavors, and immediate interaction in the case of an emergency, then a direct caregiver who is responsible for only that child is usually recommended.

(8) Pre-admission Preparation: For most students who require health technology and treatment, it is necessary to use the special education process to access related services. The process includes identification and classification as "Other Health Impaired." The assessment process for students who are classified "Other Health Impaired" can be relatively simple. In many states, it requires a

review/evaluation of educational needs, a full report from a physician which provides information about the implications of the student's illness for school participation and learning, and documentation of necessary services needed to participate successfully in school. Classification as "Other Health Impaired" does not automatically mean special education classes. It can be the avenue to provide the support necessary to participate in a regular education program.

After a student has been evaluated and classified, an Individual Education Plan (IEP) is written. For most students, decisions regarding placement and the implementation of their school program can be made at the IEP meeting. The IEP team protects the student's rights and assures that the school system is not making decisions for and without the parent/guardian and student. For students who require health technology and procedures, however, initial planning and decision-making will have to be completed before the usual IEP process.

Planning should begin while the student is in the hospital gaining medical stability. Early identification allows for a head start on planning. It affords educators the opportunity to network with other school personnel who have successfully provided educational services to similar students. It allows time for intrasystem networking, resource evaluation, building modifications, and personnel preparation. Early identification creates adequate time to determine and document specific health needs of the student in school, as well as to assist families and school personnel to secure resources for personnel training in the care of the student (Caldwell, Todaro, & Gates, 1989).

During the planning process it should be determined who is responsible for coordination and decision-making for the student. Administrative planning for this type of student is often the responsibility of the school's special education administrator. These administrators most often receive assistance from school health professionals. Guidelines developed by the staff of Project School Care at Boston Children's Hospital recommend that a health care coordinator, usually a school nurse, be selected as soon as the child is identified. This coordinator acts as liaison among the family, school, and health personnel. The Coordinator determines health needs, develops health care and emergency plans and then secures technical assistance and training (Palfrey, Haynie, Porter, & West, 1988).

In California the State Department of Education has proposed that information be completed and "synthesized" by a "medically qualified professional" defined as a credentialed school nurse, public health nurse, or physician before the IEP is written (California Department of Education, Draft Regulations, 1988).

In Louisiana, case management personnel in the health care system identify the child to the school while the child is still in the hospital. The family and program personnel network with school personnel and participate in the evaluation and planning processes (Ventilator-Assisted Care Program, 1985 b).

Securing Information

A full school health evaluation is needed for any student who requires health technology and treatment in school. Table 7.3 provides guidelines for areas which should be considered when gathering information. Not all areas of information will be necessary to consider for every student.

Transition

A crucial element of planning and evaluation is transition. If the school system does not receive early notification then a more restrictive environment may be necessary until the system is ready to provide a safe, appropriate environment. Some school systems may provide home health services in school or home instruction while gathering medical information, completing educational evaluations, and orienting school personnel. In any case, placement in home instruction or an alternative program should be time-limited and focused on transition activities.

Training is considered during transition. Both licensed and lay personnel require time to develop health plans and learn the intricacies of a student's health care. If lay persons are being trained, training is completed over time. Training begins with competence on a mannequin, supervised care to the student, and then to care without direct supervision. The family may be able to provide or assist with training.

Planning for transition to school involves the family. It is important to examine the family's needs for transition as well as the child's needs. Family members may be involved in the selection and training of caregivers. They may want to see the classroom. They may want

Table 7.3. Students Who Require Health Technology and Treatment: Screening and Assessment.

1. *Health Considerations*
   a. Health Care Plan
      Diagnosis
      Description of Condition
      Treatment/Side Effects
      Special Nutritional Requirements
      Medication/Side Effects
      Precautions
      Activity Restrictions
   b. Emergency Plan
      Warning Signs and Symptoms
      Interaction/Intervention/Emergency Reaction Time
      Emergency Contacts
      Natural Disasters
2. *Educational Considerations*
   a. Education Plan
      Level of Developmental/Educational/Vocational Function
      Physical Ability to Participate in Classroom Activities
      Educational/Communication Equipment Needs
   b. Independence in Care
      Present Level of Function
      Potential Function
   c. School Absence
      Reduced Vitality
      Time Factors
      Program Accommodations
3. *Placement Considerations*
   a. Environment
      Accessible
      Temperature Control
      Allergens
      Environmental Hazards
      Running Water
      Electrical Requirements
      Storage Area
      Private Area to Complete Procedures
   b. Personnel/Consumer Requirements
      Need for Supplemental/Related Services
      Need for Direct Care Personnel
        Licensure Required
        Training and Supervision
      Orientation/Technical Assistance
        Direct Care Personnel
        Supplemental/Related Services Personnel
        Administrators
        School Personnel
        Classmates
        Schoolmates
        PTA/Community
   c. Transportation
      Accessible
      Secure for Student
      Secure for Equipment
      Temperature Control
      Trained Personnel
      Emergency Plan

Note: From *The Community Provider's Guide: An Information Outline for Working with Children with Special Needs in the Community* (p. IV 9–10) by T. Caldwell, A. Todaro, and A. J. Gates, 1989, New Orleans, Louisiana: Children's Hospital. Reprinted with permission.

to be hired as the direct caregiver in the classroom until they are comfortable that their child will be safe in school.

Developing the IEP

The next step in the education process involves the development of the student's Individual Education Plan (IEP). This plan summarizes student functioning, as well as outlines goals and objectives, environmental modifications, and resources the student will require. At minimum, the parent/guardian and school system personnel are involved in IEP development. For the student who has special health needs, the involvement of health personnel is important. According to Caldwell, Todaro and Gates (1989), included in an IEP for students who require health technology and treatment are:

(1) Documentation of services the student needs.
(2) Documentation of who is responsible for supervising or providing for the student's special health needs.
(3) Outline of the progression to be followed in teaching the student to increase tolerance, direction of others, or completion of health procedures independently.

Placement

Placement is the final step in the initial process. Most state regulations require that each student be placed in an appropriate classroom which is within a limited age range, taught by teachers with particular certification, and in the school closest to home. The other regulations deal with LRE and the opportunity for special students to attend school with their peers.

Regulations and health variables must be considered when making placement decisions. The first decision is whether the student is stable enough to go to school. Collaboration among family members, physician, health care providers, school, and other personnel such as foster care assist to make this decision. If the student is not stable, home or hospital instruction will often be recommended. If the student is stable and participation in school is appropriate, the placement/IEP committee can examine the educational needs of the student and follow the normal regulations which affect placement. For a child living in the community it is usually not appropriate to elect

**Table 7.4. Students Who Require Health Technology and Treatment:
Recommendations for Training.**

1. Secure individualized prescriptions and protocols including warning signs and symptoms. Develop these in collaboration with parents and health care providers.
2. Begin training prior to student's return to community. Have parent observe and/ or participate in training.
3. Train at least two people so that back-up is available. Delivery of care by a consistent provider(s) is important to maintenance of student health.
4. Train all personnel who will work with the student to deal with emergency situations, i.e. bus driver, adapted physical education teacher, anyone else teaching the student. Recommend that the on-site administrator and/or secretary learn emergency procedures.
5. For a designated period, an expert (i.e. qualified professional, trained parent caregiver) should be present for continued training and on-site back-up. Length of back-up is determined by care provider's competency and comfort. It is recommended that at least five trials of procedures and emergencies with 100 percent accuracy be documented before care provider works independently.
6. Document training using individualized checklist. The trainer and parent sign the checklist after training is completed.
7. Re-checks are recommended by the trainer with timelines based on complexity of procedures and competency of care provider.
8. Training and re-checks should include recognition and implementation of emergency procedures.

Note: From *The Community Provider's Guide: An Information Outline for Working with Children with Special Needs in the Community* (p. III 2–3) by T. Caldwell, A. Todaro, and A.J. Gates, 1989, New Orleans, Louisiana: Children's Hospital. Reprinted with permission.

a hospital-based or institutional school. A student who is ventilator-assisted may attend a regular class in the neighborhood school. After a class and school have been selected, it is necessary to develop the necessary resources to support that school in the placement.

Training, Supervision, and Monitoring

Training planning must incorporate "that every professional, parent and community provider has unique skills, and the major goal of training is to expand those skills so that the professional may competently provide quality community-based care." (Pathfinders, 1989, p. 20). The steps in Table 7.4 recognize the individual needs of the child and the persons to be trained.

Louisiana resources for assistance in training include a videotape and workbook for ventilator-assisted students (Whitsel, Carlin, & Cimo, 1989), a guide for community-based program development (Caldwell, Todaro, & Gates, 1989), and a parent-oriented guidebook (Ventilator Assisted Care Program, 1985 a).

ROLES OF PERSONNEL ACROSS SYSTEMS

In school settings, the parent or guardian often becomes the liaison and coordinator of services who receives information from others, shares that information, and coordinates collaboration. The parent/ guardian provides all equipment and supplies needed for health procedures at school and coordinates with home care vendors when there is a problem with equipment. The other role is advocate and protector of the child's development. It is often the family's will and tenacity which has assured their child's attendance.

Community and school health personnel, including physicians, nurses, therapists, and vendors can assist the school in providing information, direct services and/or monitoring of overall health status. In addition, community health personnel assist with broken equipment and provide emergency treatment.

Tertiary specialists, including physicians, nurses, and therapists, are involved in intensive, acute, and rehabilitative care. In the past, they have rarely been involved in school care decisions. For the student who requires health technology and treatment, the involvement of tertiary specialists is essential. The tertiary specialists evaluate the student's ongoing need for technology, recommend the specific types of technology, and determine how the technology will be used in all community settings. Their involvement in the development of the school health care plan is crucial.

Collaboration among school, community, and tertiary health personnel has historically been limited. Communication with personnel across systems is often difficult. Ongoing collaboration and communication are key to the success of school placement for students who require health technology and treatment.

CONCLUSION

Students with health technology and treatment have the right to receive an education in the least restrictive environment. Education is one of the most difficult services to organize because of a lack of program models, inadequate resources, fear of health maintenance procedures in the school setting, and a lack of collaboration among systems. These difficulties can be managed. For youth who are medically stable, LRE is usually located at a community school where additional resources are provided. Education provides the major path to adult vocation and self-sufficiency for all youth. Students with medical technology and treatment need all aspects of a normal school day, including pre-academics, academics, (adapted) physical education, vocationally-relevant training, field trips, socialization, extracurricular activities, and more. These students require additional attention to planning, training and monitoring of health care providers. The students need to be involved in their health care programs. Families, education, and health care systems have a responsibility to work together to achieve academically-appropriate school services. LEA's and SEA's must develop models of community-based school services which fit into the context of local needs and resources.

REFERENCES

Aday, L. A., Aitken, M. J., & Wegener, D. H. (1988). *Pediatric home care: Results of a national evaluation of programs for ventilator-assisted children*. Chicago: Pluribus.

Caldwell, T., Todaro, A., & Gates, A. J. (1989). *Community provider's guide: An information outline for working with children with special needs in the community*. New Orleans, Louisiana: Children's Hospital.

Caldwell, T., Todaro, A., & Gates, A. J. (1990). Special Health Care Needs. In J. L. Bigge. *Teaching individuals with physical and multiple disabilities* (Third Edition). Columbus, Ohio: Charles E. Merrill Publishing Co., 1990.

California Department of Education. (1988). *Draft regulations*. Unpublished manuscript.

Council for Exceptional Children's Ad Hoc Committee on Medically Fragile Students (1988). *Report of the council for exceptional children's ad hoc committee on medically fragile students*. Reston, Virginia: Council for Exceptional Children.

Hochstadt, N. J. & Yost, D. M. (1989). The Health Care Child Welfare Partnership: Transitioning medically complex children to the community. *Children's Health Care, 18*(1), 4–11.

Kirkhart, K. & Gates, A. J. (1988). Home care of children assisted by high-tech supports. In H. M. Wallace, G. Ryan, & A. C. Oglesby (Eds). *Maternal and child health practices (Third Edition)*. Oakland, California: Third Party Publishing Co., 673–681.

Kirkhart, K., Steele, N. F., Pomeroy, M., Anguzza, R., French, W. & Gates, A. J. (1989). Louisiana's ventilator-assisted care program: Case management services to link tertiary with community-based care. *Children's Health Care, 17*(2), 106–111.

Louisiana Office of Special Education Services (1983). *Louisiana's law for exceptional students: Bulletin 1706, Regulations for implementation of the exceptional children's act.* (R.S. 17: 1941 et seg.)

Palfrey, J. Haynie, L. Porter, S. & West, G. (1989). *Children assisted by medical technology in educational settings. Guidelines for care.* Boston, Massachusetts: The Children's Hospital.

Public Law 94-142, November 29, 1975. House Document Room, U.S. Capitol, Washington, D.C., 20510.

Reiser, L. (1989, October). The obligation to serve: Legal sources. In Education of the handicapped and EDLAW, Inc. (Chairs), *Serving medically fragile and technology-dependent children in the 1990's.* Conference, Ft. Lauderdale, FL.

Shelton, T. L., Jeppson, E. S., & Johnson, B. H. (1987). *Family-centered care for children with special health care needs.* Washington, D.C.: Association for the Care of Children's Health.

Sirvos, Barbara. (1988). Students with special health care needs, *Teaching Exceptional Children, 20,* 40–44.

Sokoloff, S. S., Lewis, R. B., Lynch, E. W., & Murphy, D. S. (1986). *Care book of legislation and litigation related to chronically ill children.* San Diego, California: San Diego State University.

Task Force on Technology-Department Children. (1988). *Fostering home and community-based care for technology-dependent children: Report of the task force on technology-dependent children.* (Volumes 1–2), (DHHS Publication No. HCFA 88-02171). Washington, D.C.: U.S. Government Printing Office.

U.S. Congress, Office of Technology Assessment. (1987). *Technology dependent children: Hospital v. home care—A technical memorandum* (Publication No. OTA-TM-H-38). Washington, D.C.: U.S. Government Printing Office.

Ventilator-Assisted Care Program. (1985 a). *Homeward bound: resources for living at home with a chronically ill child.* New Orleans, Louisiana: Children's Hospital.

Ventilator-Assisted Care Program. (1985 b). *Training materials for educational settings.* New Orleans, Louisiana: Children's Hospital.

Vitello, S. J. (1987). School Health Services after "Tatro." *Journal of School Health, 57*(2), 77–80.

Whitsel, E., Carlin, P., & Cimo, D. (1987). *Getting it started and keeping it going: A guide for respiratory home care of the ventilator-assisted individual.* New Orleans, Louisiana: Children's Hospital.

Wood, S., Walker, D., & Gardner, J. (1986). School health practices for children with complex medical needs. *Journal of School Health, 56* (6), 215–216.

Section V
Parenting Medically Complex Children

CHAPTER 8

MEDICAL FOSTER CARE: THE FOSTER PARENTS' PERSPECTIVE

LYNN PRYBYL
THOMAS PRYBYL

INTRODUCTION

It was a warm summer day in August as my husband Tom and I
drove from our suburban home into Chicago to La Rabida Children's
Hospital (LRCH). Although we did not know it at the time this would
become an almost daily 70 mile round trip to the hospital to visit a
very special child.

Our family had been fostering infants in temporary care for about
seven years. During those seven years we cared for 29 foster children.
There was no doubt in my mind that this was a special calling for our
family. Our two children, Adam (age 15) and Diana (age 12), were
attending school all day and I had many empty hours available. Many
women look for work outside of the home at this point in their lives;
I was looking to do something that would be a blessing to others as
well as rewarding to myself and my family. Foster care seemed to be
the ideal answer for me.

Now, seven years after we had begun our foster care experience
we were about to embark on a new journey. It was June, 1986, when
a newsletter came from our foster care agency, Children's Home and
Aid Society of Illinois (CHASI), announcing a new project requiring
foster families to care for "medically complex children." I was unsure
as to what medically complex really meant. At first, it did not seem
to matter to me. I was happy taking care of young infants, helping
them to grow and develop, preparing them to go home or to an
adoptive family. However, the words "medically complex children"
seemed to stick with me for the next few days. I decided to share
what little information I had with other members of my family.

They all reacted in the same way, "no way"!

After several more days I noticed that Tom and the children were beginning to ask more and more questions about medically complex children . . . questions I could not answer. It didn't take very long for us to decide that we needed more information.

The next day I telephoned CHASI and talked with the supervisor of this new project. I was told that there were many different types of medically complex children. All had medical problems but some were "technology dependent." This meant that devices or machines were needed to assist these children's bodily functions. I was given some basic information such as the age range of the children in the project, some general medical facts, the kind of care they required and what prospective foster parents would have to do to care for these children. For example, prospective foster parents would most likely be involved with approximately eight weeks of training, and would need to house the child, equipment, a large quantity of supplies, and a home health care nurse for at least eight hours each day.

The CHASI social worker was not sure how long a medically complex child would remain in foster care but estimated that it might be as long as 1½ to 2 years. Until this point, we had only cared for children for an average of six to eight months. On the few occasions when one of our foster children stayed a year or more, it had been extremely difficult for us to say goodbye. However, I sensed the real need these medically complex children have for a home, a family and a loving environment where they could grow and experience so much of the world that was missing in their hospital room.

I was also beginning to realize at this time that we were one of the few families to express an interest in caring for these children. As it turned out we would be the first family in the project. We would be the first to help work out the many problems as well as experience the many triumphs.

The more our family discussed the possibility of caring for a medically complex child the more we felt we had to go on and obtain more information.

OUR FIRST MEETING WITH THE HEALTH CARE TEAM

The next step was for Tom and I to attend a medical staffing where we would hear about a specific child (John—a 16 month-old boy) who had been selected as a possible foster child for us.

At the staffing we were told by one of John's physicians about his diagnosis, history and prognosis. John had become ill at three months of age with severe croup. Because of John's extreme coughing, his vocal chords and epiglotus became paralyzed. He had reactive airway disease and also had a feeding problem i.e., he was prone to aspirate his food. John had a tracheostomy so that he could breathe and a gastric tube inserted into his stomach for feedings. As a result of the tracheostomy he was unable to talk.

After John's medical condition was stabilized, a decision was made to transfer him from the acute care hospital to La Rabida Children's Hospital. La Rabida Children's Hospital serves as a specialized pediatric transitional facility. In addition, LRCH and CHASI had just received a federal grant to enable a pediatric hospital and a child welfare agency to develop a program to transition medically complex children to foster care.

In addition to his medical problems John was very withdrawn and developmentally delayed. Thanks to the help of the excellent hospital staff and a foster grandparent John began to make excellent progress.

At the time of the first medical staffing John was breathing through a Shiley tracheotomy tube. He had to have a mist collar on his trach most of the day and night. He had to receive nebulizer and chest percussion treatments (CPT's) every six hours; more frequently when he was ill. John was eating chopped and pureed foods by mouth and his gastric tube was removed shortly after admission to LRCH. Several therapists were working with John to improve his fine and gross motor skills along with teaching him sign language.

The prognosis for the removal of John's trach and regaining his speech were "encouraging but unsure." This was a phrase we would hear over and over again with regard to John and other children in the project.

The social worker from the hospital shared with us a little of John's social history along with the other specific needs and responsibilities we would have to fulfill if we agreed to take him home. Because of many social problems John's biological family was unable to manage his complex medical care. As a result, John had been placed in temporary custody of the state social service agency.

If we agreed to care for John there were many tasks we would have to perform. For example, we would have to find a local pediatrician who would accept the Public Aid card for payment to supervise John's care after discharge. We would have to learn sign language and to continue to teach John how to sign. There would be the possibility of weekly visits with his biological parents. We would also be expected to continue his therapy with a variety of health care providers and to be available for medical follow-up visits when necessary. Together with the hospital social worker, we would have to develop an emergency plan with the electric, telephone and gas company and with our local police and fire department. This plan was needed in case of power outages, a phone failure or a medical emergency.

Naturally, we had many questions. For example, was John's condition so unstable that he might die in our home? We were told that John was one of the more stable children in the project but that there was still a chance, albeit small, that he could die in our care. Was it possible for John to become available for adoption and would we be considered a resource because of the racial difference? We were told that the goal at this point was to stabilize John and prepare his biological family for his return home. However, transracial adoption was a possible option in the future should the need arise. Another question we had was whether our children would be allowed to visit and learn John's care while he was hospitalized. This was agreeable to everyone as long as their visits were prearranged. Our biggest question was whether we could back out of the project once we started training. Everyone agreed that we could back out of the project at any time. Little did we know just how committed we would become in a very short period of time. When we look back now, we realize how much more we would have been willing to do to help this terrific little guy.

OUR FIRST MEETING

Suddenly, all of our questions had been asked and answered. There was only one more thing left to do . . . meet John. I grabbed my purse and a small toy we had brought for him, but I remember little else of the walk from the conference room to his room. Never before in my life had I experienced such panic, fear, anxiety and sheer excitement all at the same time. Would John like us? Would we be able to love and care for him? Were we taking on more than we could handle? I couldn't wait to hold him!

One last turn and we were in a room with two cribs. One darling little boy was sitting in a high chair watching Sesame Street when we arrived. Could this be John? As everyone passed him and went to the second crib I spotted John under the crib crawling on the floor.

His primary nurse picked him up and brought him over to meet us. From the smile on Tom's face I could tell he was in love with John at the first sight.

There in front of me was a plump little boy with empty eyes and an expressionless face. He had to be coaxed to take the small toy we brought for him, and then only after we gave it to his nurse to give to him.

I heard little else spoken in John's room that afternoon. I could not take my eyes off this small child. After the nurse placed him in his bed and he began to fall asleep I reached through the bars of the crib to gently stroke his leg. It was at this moment that my commitment was made. I knew that whether it was for two months, two years, or forever, we would be John's family.

Tom and I drove home anxious to share our thoughts and feelings with Adam and Diana. Our two older children played an active role in caring for our other foster children and we were anxious to talk about their concerns and feelings about this new child.

Our children were primarily concerned about three things. What did he look like? Was he hooked up to a lot of machines? Could they play with him? With these questions answered we decided to take two more days to think and pray about bringing John home. The vote was finally taken, and I called the social worker to say we would like to be John's foster family.

VISITING

After a week of waiting with no word, and being a very impatient person, I called CHASI to find out if we could start visiting John to develop a relationship with him before we began learning his medical care. From my readings, I knew that these children only trusted one or two people to change their trachs. I hoped that Tom and I would gain his trust before we would actually have to change the trach.

I also knew that John was extremely attached to his primary care nurse and to his foster (volunteer) grandfather. Somehow our family would also have to become important to him; this seemed possible only through frequent visiting.

Several days later we were given permission to visit John whenever we wanted to for the month of November. Our formal training was to begin in December. My first day of visiting arrived and I could barely contain my excitement. I drove Adam and Diana to school at

7:30 a.m. and headed for the hospital. My excitement was allowed to cool for almost two hours as I sat in morning rush hour traffic. I finally arrived at the hospital carrying my bag of specially selected toys and books and headed for John's room.

John was already dressed and had just finished breakfast when I arrived. He was playing with his foster grandfather, Harry, a man who was one of John's most valued and loved caregivers.

Because I knew nothing about trach care, I was only permitted to stay in John's room with him and play on a matt on the floor. At first, John seemed to be fearful of the toys I had brought and his face remained empty and expressionless. After an hour, I discovered by accident the real key to pleasing this little boy. He loved to have someone sing to him—he loved music. I started with row, row, row your boat and proceeded to sing every song, nursery rhyme and hymn I knew. Each visit, for the next week or so, John fell asleep with his head on my chest as I sang on and on.

During the first week of visiting I took each of our children to visit at different times so as not to over-stimulate John with too many new faces. Adam and Diana were both pleasantly surprised at his mobility and the fact that he was not tethered to a machine. They were disappointed in John's seeming unwillingness to relate to his soon to be foster brother and sister. Fortunately, this was only temporary. Adam and Diana shifted into high gear and introduced John and his roommate to basketball, hospital room style, and to a tape recorder. Diana taught them hand clapping and finger play songs. It was terrific to see how the children responded.

It was difficult being at the hospital with John and feeling like I was in the way. I also became very aware of how much I didn't know about caring for him. One lunch hour he began to choke on some food and I had to run to get help. I also felt that John was not following his normal routine on the days I was there. When John's nurses recommended that Tom and I start our training earlier than planned I was elated.

TRAINING BEGINS

Tom and I were told we would need approximately nine two-hour trainings sessions. We chose Wednesdays, Tom's day off, as our training day so that we could both be there at the same time. We also sat down as a family and worked out our weekly schedule for hospital training and visits.

Our training sessions progressed faster than anticipated and by the first of January we were able to assume almost full care of John while we were in the hospital.

We learned a great deal about John's care throughout our training. We learned John's nutritional program and how to feed him. The hospital staff patiently taught us how to suction, clean and change his trach and trach ties. They stood by to help whenever it was necessary. They gave us specific instructions in cardiopulmonary resuscitation, what to do if he was choking and information on other problems and emergency situations. The respiratory therapist showed us how to adjust his equipment, give nebulizer treatments and chest percussion treatments. We were trained to administer his medication and to look for side effects. We also learned all aspects of his personal care and hygiene. More than anything else, the hours and hours of patient supervised care and conversations with the staff at LRCH made our job so much easier.

Of particular help was being able to sit in on John's play group and watching him interact with other children and with his foster grandfather. The help we received from John's developmental and his speech and language therapists was of tremendous assistance. Most important were the hours of caring conversation I shared with John's primary care nurse, Bessie, and other members of the nursing staff. They made it easier to really get to know, love and understand this terrific child.

It had been two months since the first time we saw John and it was getting harder and harder to be away from him. Tom found his visits on Wednesdays, to change John's trach, stretching into three and four hour stays. John was having difficulties too. He cried and tantrumed whenever we had to leave. This did not help us, but it showed the hospital staff just how well he was bonding to our family. When John unselfishly shared a respiratory virus with me, and I was unable to visit for eight days, I was overwhelmed from the anxiety of separation. We knew the day was drawing nearer for John's discharge and we were all more than ready.

PLANNING THE TRANSITION TO HOME CARE

At long last a discharge meeting was scheduled and our last two weeks of training were set. Everything was scheduled so that the transition to home care would be gradual and incremental. First, I was scheduled to care for John over a 24 hour period in the hospital. This was extremely informative and helpful. Little did I know then that two years down the road I would be able to give nebulizer treatments in the dark and still not be used to a child who starts his day at 5 a.m.

Three days later John came home on an eight hour pass. This proved to be an invaluable learning experience. This was John's first experience outside the hospital environment and we immediately recognized the need to limit the area available to him. For example, John was not aware of the dangers in the kitchen, especially now since food did not come already prepared on a tray but had to be cooked. He did not understand that stairs had depth, that plants were not food and that some things could fall over on top of him when pushed.

Two days after our eight hour pass a 24 hour pass was scheduled. John's home equipment, which was slightly different from what was used in the hospital, did not work properly. We also had our first opportunity to deal with a plugged airway. Because John was going back to the hospital for one day, this gave us a chance to work out these equipment problems with our vendor. This 24 hour pass also gave us our first experience with home health nursing care and showed us just how much family routine was going to be changed.

Most memorable of all was how disappointed and hurt we felt when we returned John to the hospital the next morning only to find him happy to be back. He settled right into his room and ignored us completely. I really wondered if this was going to work out.

A day later we brought John home for the weekend on a 48 hour pass. Things were now going more smoothly. John's new equipment worked well, the home health nurse came and abided by our house rules, Adam and Diana supplied endless hours of entertainment in a two room gated-off area, and we all began to feel good about being a family. There was only one problem. I was exhausted from trying to do all the work myself. I felt both relieved and guilty when I returned John to the hospital on Monday morning. All I could think about was going home and getting some sleep. This time the guilt increased even more when John did not want to stay in the hospital.

The next morning I was at the hospital again, this time to accompany the nurse and John to visit an ear, nose and throat specialist at another hospital. I quickly learned that a 9 a.m. appointment could mean not leaving the clinic until 1 or 2 in the afternoon. One more lesson was learned this day. Come prepared with food and toys to occupy a child for a lengthy period of time.

I also realized that for these specialty clinic appointments I needed more information about John's medical history and a greater familiarity with medical terminology. When I asked the ENT doctor about John's prognosis his answers were very vague. I also felt extremely disappointed because John's condition had not changed or improved in the past six months.

GETTING READY AT HOME

While all this was going on at the hospital, there were many other arrangements to make at home.

First, I strongly recommend obtaining books from your local library on general home health care. These provided me with definitions of terms and treatments hospital staff and therapists often use. A good medical dictionary is also a necessity. Sometimes your pediatrician will give you one that he is no longer using.

Soon after we decided to care for John a representative from the State of Illinois, Division of Services for Crippled Children (DSCC), visited our home to assist us in developing a home care plan and provide funding for various home health services. The DSCC representative also informed us how DSCC could help in locating equipment vendors and home health nursing agencies. Since we lived so far away from LRCH she was also able to help us locate local medical caregivers who would accept Public Aid funding. This was not as easy as it seems. Finding physicians with experience treating problems such as John's who would also accept Public Aid funding was one of our most difficult and challenging problems.

We found that it is important for foster parents to be assertive and forthright about their foster child's care when dealing with new physicians or other health care providers. After all, we spent hours learning about John's care from very qualified people. The care plan and discharge plans were developed because they worked well for John. Be sure that these techniques are not tossed aside by a physician or health care providers who don't have the same long-term relationship with the child as you or the previous health care providers.

After more than a year of changing pediatricians and several serious respiratory illnesses we decided to forego the use of the Public Aid card and take John to our own pediatrician whom we trusted and respected. This proved to be one of the best decisions we made in caring for John.

The choice of an equipment and supply vendor is critical. Because we had an excellent experience with a vendor in our area and had developed a good working relationship with one of their respiratory therapists, we asked to work with them again. This respiratory therapist was invaluable in helping us set-up, maintain and use our apnea monitor, portable and stationery suction machines, compressor, mist collar, oxygen and nebulizer equipment. If at all possible it is helpful to develop a working relationship with one person within the equipment and supply company that you deal with. This person can be an invaluable source of support and assistance.

A major problem for us was getting the supplies we needed. After John had been home for approximately six weeks we were able to work out a list of supplies we would need monthly. The supply company was given a copy of these items on several occasions but they never seemed to have the correct amount or correct sizes available when I called to order. After six months of wrong orders or back orders we solved this problem by keeping our own small stock for emergency use.

Fortunately, the nursing agency was better organized than the equipment vendors. At the outset, we explained to the nursing personnel that we wanted to be responsible for John's care when Tom and I were in the home. We would ask the nurse for assistance or advice if we needed it, but wanted them to understand that they were there primarily as an emergency back-up. Of course, when we were not in the home they would be totally responsible for John's care.

This arrangement worked for some nurses and not for others. Our two primary care nurses abided by our request and became respected additions to our family. Most of the problems occurred with temporary relief or substitute nurses who were either unwilling to do things our way or were too inexperienced.

For example, it didn't take us too long to learn that there was a difference between trach care *certified* and trach care *experienced*. One evening, as Tom and I were preparing to go out with friends for dinner, I asked the substitute nurse if he had trach experience. He replied "Yes I do. I have observed one being changed once." Needless to say, Tom and I did not leave home that evening.

Nursing care in the home can be a positive experience if all the ground rules are set-up ahead of time. Thanks to our social worker, we were able to by-pass many of the problems other families have experienced by putting together a small notebook of house rules which each nurse was asked to read either at orientation or before starting work with us. This notebook contained such rules as where to park their car, which rooms of the house were available for their use, what kitchen equipment and utensils could be used, rules for use of the telephone and television, along with our care plan for John and appropriate dress (we requested that nurses wear uniforms while on duty). These clearly presented rules helped prevent many problems and made our relationship with the home health nurses much easier.

We found it particularly helpful to convert a fifth bedroom, adjacent to John's room, into a study/play area for our nursing staff. This room had an intercom directly to John's room, a desk, television, telephone, and toys. This provided the nurse with her own room thereby limiting the intrusion of nursing staff into our home.

The hours of conversation with our social worker were invaluable. She helped us remember how important it was to meet the needs of all of our family members. She also helped us work on issues surrounding the visits of John's biological parents and she was always available to help with problems as they came up.

There were many details to arrange in those frantic days before John came home. This included setting up appointments with his new pediatrician, re-scheduling appointments with the ear, nose and throat specialist, and getting an appointment for John to be evaluated by the local school district so that he could participate in a 0-3 developmental program.

GOING HOME

Three months after first meeting John, and seven months since our decision to become involved in this project, the discharge day finally arrived. Tom and I had been gradually taking John's personal belongings home so that all we had to carry home was John.

As we left there was a slight fear that we might fail and the realization that we were not bringing him back to the hospital the next day. I remember feeling this day was rather anticlimatic after all the preparations. Nonetheless, we were still very excited. After leaving the hospital our first activity was to pick up Adam and Diana from school. Our family was now complete.

SETTLING IN

The first days still remain a blur of incredible activity. Many people were in and out of our home e.g., social workers, therapists, nurses, supervisors, etc.

We needed to develop a routine for John's medical and physical care, equipment maintenance, supply ordering, therapies, school, family and church activities. It wasn't long before we all sensed the need for some changes and adjustments.

We decided that the best way to do this was for each of us to make a list of our activities in the order of their importance. It soon became evident that a few activities and responsibilities, such as teaching church youth groups, would have to be temporarily shelved and that we needed to utilize our nursing care hours in a more practical way.

At first, it was extremely reassuring to have a nurse with John and I during the daytime hours. However, I began to see the need to have her there when I needed to be out. John had pulled his trach out several times, had been ill and in respiratory distress, had fallen down more than once and I felt comfortable with our emergency plans and knew they worked. I had no doubt about my abilities to cope with John, what I needed most was a nurse to care for John when I needed to be out of the home. For instance, in the middle of winter our nurse started one-half hour before I needed to drive our other children to school. I would then do my grocery shopping and other errands and be home in time to feed John lunch. Similarly, I arranged the nursing schedule so that several days during the week they started one-half hour before I picked the children up from school and stayed with John while we attended church activities. It was also helpful to schedule doctors' appointments and parental visits when the nurse was able to accompany us. This provided me with freedom to talk with John's doctors. While in the car the nurse attended to his trach care so that I did not have to stop.

Because Adam and Diana have been so willing to help with John's medical care Tom and I felt it was a good idea to spend one evening a week just with them. This became our regular Friday date night. Sometimes we would all go out together, or Tom and I would each take one of the children for a one-on-one evening. On the few occasions when Adam and Diana were busy with friends Tom and I would go out alone.

It took at least 8 to 12 weeks to set up our schedule and begin functioning within it. One thing we learned early on was to be very flexible and to accept the circumstances we could not change. Often schedules had to be changed at a moment's notice. For example, when John became ill, Tom or I would always be home with him. Most of our friends were very understanding about last minute changes in our plans. At the same time, we requested that people not visit us if they were ill. We all continued to remind ourselves that this was only a temporary situation and John's health and mobility would improve with time . . . and it did.

We also learned to expect the unexpected. One evening around midnight John spiked a temperature of 105° and had difficulty breathing. The secretions from his trach had turned yellow (indicating an infection) and we were off to our local emergency room. Fortunately, we always carried a bag of medical supplies with us. When we arrived at the local emergency room, they had no suction catheters small enough to clean out his trach. It would have taken 10 to 15 minutes for them to get one from the medical supply room . . . a long time for a choking child to wait. We supplied the catheter from our bag of medical supplies. Again, an important problem had surfaced. Many doctors in smaller community hospitals are not familiar or equipped to handle medically complex children.

ABSOLUTE JOYS

Amidst all of the medical care and therapy are hours of absolute joy. It is extremely rewarding to be able to observe, and be part of, the physical improvement and developmental accomplishments of children. The sheer delight on John's face and the disappearance of those empty expressionless eyes are what make this specialized foster care experience so rewarding. After all, a child who awakens you every morning between four and five o'clock is not always welcome. However, if you add a jump on your bed, an Eskimo kiss and some newly acquired sign language your heart melts and you find the energy to get out of bed. Grocery shopping, church, and park, bowling, basketball games, and the movies all take on a new meaning when you are with a child who has never been there before. You begin to look for, and encourage, all of those things a child can do and overlook those things he cannot. Giving love, sharing love and accepting love are the true joys of life.

NEW CHALLENGES

Just as we learned to expect the unexpected, we now have learned that new challenges will face us every day. Medical needs increase, decrease and sometimes completely change. Schooling for a medically complex child brings parents and child into a whole new world. Foster parents must know the child's educational rights and be willing to advocate for the child.

Other helpful hints include keeping a daily journal and taking pictures. Obtain as much previous family medical history as well as copies of your child's medical records. Keep these handy. Everyone treating your child will need this information. This helps to avoid the need for unnecessary treatment or guesswork. Speak with your neighbors and/or friends ahead of time and explain the foster child's special needs and condition. With knowledge comes understanding.

CONCLUSION

The hum of the machines in John's room is gone. All that remains is the gentle, consistent breathing of a sleeping three-year-old little boy.

It has been two years now since John came home. There have been a few valleys to walk through but an endless number of mountain top experiences.

We have grown in faith, family unity and purpose, and in our ability to love unconditionally and share our time and talents unselfishly.

Would we change anything about our involvement in the project? Probably. Would we do it again? Definitely!

CHAPTER 9

THE ADOPTION EXPERIENCE

JUDITH GEISSLER
EVAN GEISSLER

FOREWORD

Judith and Evan Geissler were approved for an adoptive placement
of a special needs child by the Illinois Department of Children and
Family Services in the fall of 1973. Their application was in response
to an article about "Timmie," an infant with severe spina bifida and
hydrocephalus for whom an adoptive resource was being sought,
which appeared in the Chicago Sun Times article "Sunday's Child."
Timmie met his new family for the first time when he was eight months
old and was placed in their home after a period of emotional preparation and medical stabilization. The following is their story.

INTRODUCTION

"Happiness is a state of mind." "You are only as old as you feel."
"Beauty is only skin deep." These phrases allow us to challenge the
provincial ideas that constantly bombard us about our attitudes, am-
bitions, and acceptance of others. Our idea of what is a complex
problem or condition is balanced by our overall perception and values. Ultimately, our adopted son became our child and not a child
with multiple medical problems.

Everyone of us is different, and if we live long enough, our differences are a matter of degree, not type. Living with these exaggerated degrees of our human frailty is the price we pay for having
a medically complex child.

153

ORIENTATION TO PARENTHOOD

Most people think that their "normal child" will grow up to be normal. We wonder if it is their faith in what they perceive to be the usual course of things. Sometimes when accidents happen or problems develop, it may be harder for them to cope with the situation because they are ill prepared for this departure from the norm. When we chose a handicapped child we were prepared to deal with his peculiar problems—it became our overall orientation to parenting.

"Why in the world would anyone want a handicapped child?" We heard phrases like "challenged" and "medically complex" about a child with whom we were developing a profound attachment. We heard this many times and had our motivations questioned constantly.

At the time we were two people who were basically happy with ourselves who wanted to share our lives with somebody who desperately needed a nurturing family. By our own standards we were successful and we wanted to commit our energies to helping a child become successful by his own standards. Another strong value that we held was the inherent right of individuals to benefit from the burgeoning technology abounding in the United States.

OUR PERSONAL HISTORIES

Success and happiness are not static conditions. Politicians call it a process which is measured only by our ability. We both lost a parent when we were young. We both felt those losses deeply. We also enjoyed the love and commitment of those who remained as a presence in our lives, who tried to soften those losses for us. Perhaps that is one reason why we both wanted to make up that loss to someone else. We understood those feelings very well.

THE ADOPTION EXPERIENCE

However unique we may be, we are not unique in adopting. Our son is in a special school and in his class of eight, five of the students are adopted. It is surprising how many people are adopted or who know someone who is adopted. Adoption is like hypertension. Before you have it, only unlucky or genetically inferior people have it. Once you or a good friend or family member gets it, then some of the most gifted, kind and pleasant people also have the same condition.

Having an adopted child is much like having a biological child. You have the same hopes and fears. Some days they make you feel pride and happiness. Other days they make you wonder if you will ever survive the parenting process. We have an adopted son and a biological daughter. They seem to be good for each other. They argue like all siblings usually do. We try to share our time in a fair manner with each of our children and give them love and affection. Family events center around mutual and individual interests. Our son enjoys watching our daughter play basketball, and she cheers him on at the Special Olympics. They accept their differences and appreciate each others gifts.

PREPARATION FOR ADOPTION

When we decided to adopt a handicapped child, the next question was should we adopt a child with a single or multiple handicaps? We also wondered whether our first child should be adopted or biological. After prayerful consideration, we came to the conclusion that in the total picture it really didn't matter.

Consequently, we started to explore our adoption options by contacting the state agency. This occurred rather quickly after seeing our son's story in the local paper and experiencing a strong positive reaction to him.

We were fortunate in being assigned a case worker who was genuinely concerned about finding appropriate homes for her clients. Before discussing any particular children, considerable time was spent assessing our needs and abilities. We came to realize that adoption is not one-sided. Parents don't only adopt children—children also adopt parents, even though they may not be as active in the decision making. Needs are satisfied on both sides.

We utilized the adoption process to discuss the complex issues involved both with our worker and amongst ourselves. We had to make a decision regarding our capacity to accept a child who might not walk or be toilet trained. This was a serious and a thoughtful time for us. When we felt certain that we wished to proceed we began focusing more specifically on Timmie and less on the broader issues of adoption which we now grasped.

OUR SON IS PLACED

Timmie was born with an open spine that was surgically closed shortly after birth. He also had a tube in his head to drain excess fluid causing

hydrocephalus. This fluid problem can cause seizures, learning difficulties and/or retardation. His eyes often moved rapidly from side
to side which we understood would affect his vision.

After birth, when Tim was medically ready for discharge, he was
placed in a foster home. He was eight months old when we were first
introduced to him by his foster parents. At the time he could not sit,
roll, move his left arm or either leg. What he could do was eat,
breathe on his own and smile! He had just been released from the
hospital after one of his many surgeries. Between these surgeries he
was living in this loving foster home with two parents, well informed
of his medical needs. Early on Timmie had lots of love from them,
their three sons and the family dog who provided much stimulation
and support for him. His foster parents reminded us that he was
basically healthy except for his handicaps. Surgeries aside, he was
rarely sick during his first year of life.

We left their home feeling very encouraged and excited. However,
there were still many unanswered questions. We decided to solicit
more information from the medical community. As with many medical prognoses, very few consultants agreed. Some of the doctors and
nurses thought we were crazy and actively discouraged us. However,
most were neutral enough to realize that the decision was ours alone.
We asked our families for their support and prayers so that we would
make the right decision.

Ultimately, we concluded that the medical facts were not the issue.
The decision to build a family is based on love and trust in the future.
We knew we loved Timmie and he seemed to respond to us. We were
convinced that the medical hurdles we would face in the future could
be coped with through the strengths in our family. The only thing
left to do was finalize the adoption.

OUR LIFE TOGETHER

Our first year together was such a wonder and mixture of joy and
sadness. Since we had not elicited our families' advice about adopting
a medically complex child, we were delighted at how enthusiastically
he was accepted. The times he had to go back into the hospital, while
sobering and sad, were punctuated by joyful celebrations, when he
returned home, by family and friends. He could not sit up without
help nor could he crawl with the one arm he could actively move.
Therefore, we bought several types of crawling boards until we found

one with which he could move. He could only crawl on the kitchen floor where there wasn't any carpet. However, he wasn't used to moving himself around. Since he loved to eat we set up a trail of Cheerios on the floor to give him the incentive to crawl which he did most successfully.

The second year we moved to an apartment with a swimming pool. We found that our son could sit on the first step in the pool with the water to help him balance. A swimming instructor we found to work with him subsequently became a close personal friend of ours. Our daughter Gina was born that same year. While Timmie learned to swim she learned to crawl. Tim could swim but on land he could barely crawl with his arms. It was clear that he would never have the use of his legs. Since Tim was the role model for Gina, she learned to crawl on her hands and feet with her rear end up in the air. It was ironic the way this developed since it required more strength and coordination than using hands and knees.

LIFE GOES ON

As time went by Tim seemed to bring out the best in most of the people we encountered. He paved the way in our church by becoming the first wheelchair camper. A supportive camp director eased the way for everyone challenged by this event. A full time companion/ aid was engaged to take care of Tim's physical needs. The nurse assisted with his bowel and bladder problems. His camp activity was restricted because he could not wheel around the camp. However, the summer program had a choir camp which allowed him to partic- ipate with all the other choir members. All were amazed when he swam during his free time!

Camp has been a blessing for all of us. Everyone seems to accom- modate to his participation and are creative in solutions to some of the obvious barriers that arise. One summer as Tim was being pushed by an aid for a play activity his wheel hit a hole and he went sprawling. A broken leg, which stuck straight out for months, was the result. With all of this Tim has gone every year except last summer when he underwent a spinal fusion.

Another example of best laid plans going awry involved the Geissler "Zoo." When we were finally settled in our home our children were 8 and 6 years old. We felt it was time to get a puppy. Luckily puppies always seem to be born to dogs of extended family members so our

kids picked out an adorable ball of friendly fur. It was a special joy
for Tim to hold the "Teddy" in his lap. Over time Teddy grew into
a giant bear and being too big for laps, Tim decided that he liked
cats. Eventually, Gina trained Teddy to become a therapy dog visiting
hospitals and nursing homes. Tim was made aware of the service dogs
utilized for companionship and aid to handicapped individuals. These
dogs can pull wheelchairs up hills, carry articles like groceries or
books. Picking up the phone and opening doors is also part of their
repertoire. Was Tim interested? Not a bit. We finally got him a small
cat and they get along fine.

We periodically attended parent groups for parents of children with
special needs. While these were helpful we found that we did not
carry the same anger and guilt as birth parents who ultimately must
adjust to not having the "wished for" child. Sometimes their resent-
ments were directed at us and this was a reminder of how stressful
coping with this situation can be.

THE EDUCATIONAL SYSTEM

Tim has attended a special school for handicapped children through
the years. Typically, he received therapy for his physical and speech
problems on a regular basis. He is able to see out of only one eye at
a time and requires glasses. While he can read; he prefers television.
He, as always, swam and for the last three years prior to his spinal
fusion, participated in the Cancer Society Swim-a-Thon.

While participating in a special program in grammar school, Tim
got progressively heavier. Eventually a lift was installed in the school
bus. When he reached the fourth grade he was the first handicapped
child to mainstream part-time at a regular school near his special
school. Because of his learning problems and physical needs he spent
only half a day being mainstreamed.

The sixth grade Christmas Program was a special memory for our
family. Tim was Santa and his wheelchair was his sled. Eight of his
classmates were the reindeer. We cried with joy watching him being
pulled by his classmates. He was truly accepted as "one of the kids"
and they were certainly creative in their expression of that fact.

His grammar school years brought many changes. He required
more space and we had to physically alter our home to accommodate
him. This included a lift to get him into our home since it is not ranch
style. A special shower room was also built. When he became too

big and too weak to transfer to a car we purchased a van with a special lift to transport us. The fact that never changed was his bladder and bowel incontinence. By using medication, we could get by with three or four changes a day.

Locomotion has been an ongoing issue since we utilized the crawling board and cheerios. Through the years we were unable to find other forms of movement with few exceptions. We tried all sorts of hand propelled and electric tricycles, wagons, motorcycles and assorted vehicles, none of which worked. Tim seemed to lack the strength, balance or coordination to use most of our discoveries or adaptations. During his early school years he rowed around school with a rowcar we found. Around fifth grade we found the perfect solution. An all-terrain vehicle, battery operated with two tank-like treads, high back seat and equipped with a seat belt answered our prayers. Tim could control this vehicle with a joy stick which required only one hand. It could even go in reverse. To our surprise he never used this very much and always seemed to be happier in his wheelchair.

Periodically, our son has missed school for surgeries to replace his shunt when it malfunctioned. Since he cannot stand on his own, we had a standing frame built for him. When he became too big for standing frames a special wheelchair was obtained that allowed him to stand. The doctors felt that standing was essential for him despite his inability to walk. By this time we found the parent groups at school more useful. They all seemed to accept themselves and their children and time was spent helping and supporting one another.

ADOLESCENCE

When Tim entered high school two major changes occurred simultaneously. He returned to a special school program full time and he really grew physically. His chest size approached that of an adult while his legs and waist remained small due to his paralysis. He developed a severe and painful curvature at the base of his spine due to pressure from the increased weight of his trunk. A special spinal fusion was needed which was a two stage process. The first surgery which was through the back occurred the day before his fifteenth birthday.

This past summer was our worst summer in dealing with Tim's handicaps. He lost what independence he had gained due to his post-surgical condition. He cannot sit without help. A body brace must be worn for 12–18 months so he cannot twist his trunk or lay on his stomach. Worst of all, he cannot swim. Timing is everything and so Tim picked this summer to start his teenage rebellion against his parents. We saw this as slowing his recovery while he saw it as asserting his will and authority. Fortunately he has healed enough to be able to return to school. We are struggling through and look forward to the time when we are past the worst.

THE HEALTH CARE ENVIRONMENT

No discussion of our experience with medically complexity would be complete without attention to the issue of health care. Overall, the doctors and nurses we have met have been caring and talented. They labor under an ever increasing burden of bureaucracy and the constant threat of malpractice. The growth of technology has fostered unrealistic hopes and has fragmented care. Technicians, therapists and social workers are all part of the care that is needed. All of these human beings are under constant stress and "burnout" affects us all. The cost is emotional as well as monetary. The ripples extend into the very fabric of our society. Only time will tell if society accepts our handicapped children as worthy resources.

THE FUTURE

Tim will never be able to live independently. He will never drive and will require help with his finances. He has two and one half years of high school remaining. Then we hope that he can enter a three year transition program until he is twenty-one. Since he loves to meet and talk with people and is very outgoing we hope that he will be able to get a job. We feel there is a job out there for him somewhere. The biggest hurdles will be housing and transportation. Assistance with his dressing and toilet necessities will always be required. We remain hopeful which has been our strength through the years.

Yes, there are those who think we are crazy. Others try to make us out to be saints. The truth is that we are neither. We are simply two people who have been blessed with two children, one by adoption and the other by biological means. Would we do it again? Of course! Absolutely! But we do relate to Charlie Brown's saying: "Why is having fun always so much work?"

Section VI
Innovative Models of Specialized Care

CHAPTER 10

MEDICAL FOSTER CARE FOR ABUSED AND NEGLECTED CHILDREN

J. M. WHITWORTH
PATRICIA H. FOSTER

INTRODUCTION

> And he who gives a child a treat
> Makes joy bells ring in Heaven's street.
> But he who gives a child a home
> Builds palaces in Kingdom come . . .

> John Masefield, *The Everlasting Mercy*

The Medical Foster Care (MFC) program is a model developed by the Children's Crisis Center, Inc., Jacksonville, Florida, in response to needs first identified by our Multidisciplinary Child Protection Team program in 1978. A significant number of abused and neglected children were needlessly being boarded in hospitals because their medical demands could not be met by their biologic parents or in traditional foster care placement. In addition, many of the biologic parents had the capability of learning to meet the needs of the child but were not afforded the opportunity in a traditional medical or social service setting. A system was developed in which temporary placement in foster care with a Registered Nurse was the key element. In this model, the nurse foster parent is responsible for assessing the health status of the child, providing nursing care, administering medications and prescribed treatments. More importantly, the nurse is given the responsibility of teaching and providing a role model for the biologic parent as well as evaluating progress in a plan leading to the reunification of the family.

This model was developed to meet the needs of abused or neglected children with health problems in whom acuity had decreased below levels requiring an in-patient facility but were beyond the ability of the family, extended family or foster care system. Typical foster families are not equipped or legally qualified to perform the daily assessment, treatment and evaluation of medically fragile children. Likewise dysfunctional biologic families are often incapable of absorbing the stress of even the least complex medical care challenge without intensive training, support and supervision. Long term placement of a child in an institutional environment is not a viable alternative because it places the child at risk for psychological problems, developmental delay and the further withdrawal of biologic parents (Foster & Whitworth, 1986). With the pressure for health care cost containment combined with the increasing demands on the entire health care system related to cases of Acquired Immune Deficiency Syndrome (AIDS), new alternatives to hospitalization are being sought (Gurdin & Anderson, 1987; Tourse & Gundersen, 1988). Similarly the challenge of furnishing care for cocaine affected babies and finding innovative approaches for babies who fail to thrive continue to tax existing systems.

The MFC model offers an approach to reduce inappropriate hospitalization of children and reduce the length of foster care placement. These goals are attained through intensive intervention with children in foster care and with their biologic parents.

The Multidisciplinary Child Protection Team was developed to assist Child Protective Services (CPS) agencies in investigation, assessment and case planning for child abuse and neglect cases. In this process, there is a continuing opportunity to identify gaps in community resources and, since the team is a semi-independent body, to act in an advocacy role for the development of new services. (Whitworth, Lanier, Skinner & Lund, 1981). One such challenge was presented by the abused or neglected child in whom medical needs and social service needs placed it in a special category beyond the capabilities of existing systems. The classically defined foster care system and medical care system left little alternative to long-term, inappropriate hospitalization. This realization was the reason for the genesis of our medical foster care concept. Initial funding was provided by a Department of Health and Human Services Federal Grant #90-CA-0932, with continuation of the program through state and local resources.

From a conceptual standpoint, we felt that several new approaches were critical. First, foster parents have generally been viewed as part of the client system rather than part of a therapeutic team. The interaction between the foster parent and biologic parent is either limited or non-existent so that a potential source of support, modeling, training, and advocacy for the biologic parent is lost. Nurses are ideally suited to accepting a role of professional responsibility as foster parents for abused or neglected children with acute health problems. Furthermore, the professional nurse/client relationship is far less threatening to the self-concept of a mother whose child requires care that she is unable to provide.

The nurse's position of authority and respect allows the biologic mother to maintain her self-esteem while listening to the advice of a nurse rather than another parent without professional credentials.

Case flow to the Medical Foster Care (MFC) program in our scheme was directed through the Multidisciplinary Child Protection Team to assure that each case was evaluated by all professionals involved and to assure that all more traditional avenues had been considered. Referrals to the team generally came from CPS sources but were also received from medical care facilities. Once the (MFC) program was determined to be a viable alternative for the child and family, a referral was made to the MFC staff for assessment of eligibility for the program.

PROFESSIONAL STAFF

The professional staff of the MFC model consist of a team headed by a medical director, with a MFC coordinator, a foster care case manager, a clinical psychologist on a contractual basis and a clinical nurse specialist. The medical director is a pediatrician with a working knowledge of the handicapping conditions which may result from abuse or neglect. The role of this individual is to coordinate and assist in correlation of information from treatment resources to assist in the overall plans for the client. In our program, the medical director also provided emergency consultations for clients and MFC foster parents when needed.

The MFC coordinator may have a background in nursing or social work but must be knowledgeable of community resources, the pediatric and social work community as well as the court system. If the MFC coordinator is trained in social work, then the staff should include a clinical nurse specialist with experience in family and community health nursing who can assist in the initial assessment of each child, identify problems, develop a nursing care plan and participate in the ongoing evaluation of children in the program. The MFC coordinator schedules preplacement activities including staffings, MFC foster family briefing, preplacement meeting with biologic parents, and records the case plan. The MFC coordinator is responsible for supervising the case management, scheduling monthly MFC foster parent meetings, distributing the subsidy for professional nursing care, and coordinating the discharge planning.

The foster care case manager participates in preplacement staffings and placement procedures to assist in the formulation of the case plan. Ideally, the foster care case manager has a case load that is limited to medical foster care children. This person is responsible to the court for judicial correspondence including documentation of the written Performance Agreement, review and evaluation. The foster care case manager makes periodic visits on a monthly basis to both medical foster children and biological parents and furnishes documentation to the MFC coordinator and the professional team.

The clinical psychologist plays a critical role in providing psychological support and evaluation of the biological parents and acts as their advocate in the deliberations of the team. This role assures that biologic parents are part of the treatment plan. The psychologist offers these parents the opportunity to deal therapeutically with some of their own reactions to the demands of the social, legal, and health care systems while their children respond to the benefits of alternative placement. The psychologist also plays an important role in the process of reunification of families. The psychologist, through ongoing counseling and evaluation of biologic parents, provides evidence to assure the team that the biologic parent is adequately progressing in the development of parenting skills and is appropriate to resume parenting responsibilities.

PROCESS AND ELIGIBILITY

Children referred for the MFC program in this system were generally adjudicated dependent by the court due to a primary diagnosis of abuse or neglect, and evaluation for medical foster care was determined to be the best alternative for placement under the adjudication order. Return to the biologic family was controlled not only by the team but also by the court. Although not common in our program, voluntary placement has been used successfully by others (Karniski, Van Buren & Cupoli, 1986). In the case of voluntary placement, a

Table 10.1. Medical Foster Care Case Flow.

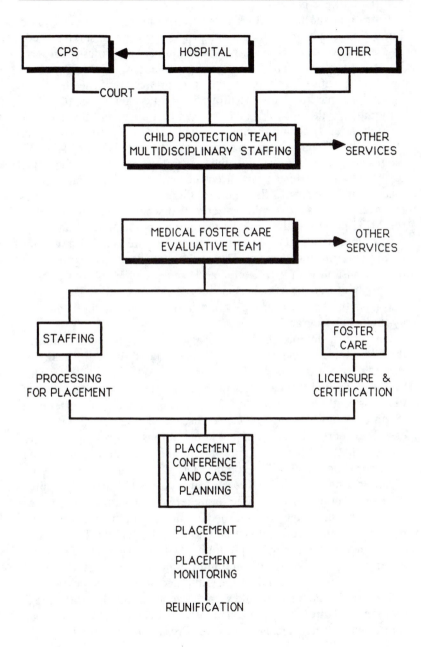

clear contractual arrangement needs to exist between the program and the biologic parents.

Entry into the MFC program is accessed by referral to the Child Protection Team for staffing. This process provides a service needs assessment for a broad spectrum of community and professional services for the client. The assessment provided by the MFC staff is program specific and addresses the appropriateness of the client and his biologic parent(s) for the program. To be eligible for the MFC program, a child must also meet criteria that document the need for nursing care. The multidisciplinary team assess the child's medical status, identify the nursing care needs and the capability of the biologic family. In concert with the medical assessment by the MFC team, the district foster care licensure and placement unit reviews placement resources to determine if there are other existing placement alternatives. It should be noted that when a child is placed in the MFC program, the biologic family enters the traditional foster care system simultaneously with the same requirements as any other family entering that system. The traditional foster care system has the responsibility for certification and licensure of MFC homes, basic foster parent training as well as monitoring all placements. This agency also pays the basic foster care financial rate which is supplemented by the MFC program.

One critical feature of the MFC assessment is the application of the Child Care Assessment Tool (CCAT) to determine the acuity of care needed for each child (Davis, Foster & Whitworth, 1984). This tool was adapted from another rating instrument that was developed to assess needs and board rates of handicapped children in foster care (Shah & Poulos, 1974). The CCAT lists child care needs in the categories of personal care, nursing interventions and psychosocial responses that are checked if appropriate and rated on a scale of one to three. (For copies of the complex CCAT write to the authors.)

The scoring yields three levels of care. At Level I, a child requires the same amount of care, time and energy as would another foster child of the same age without medical or developmental problems. Because nursing care is not justified, a dependent child with this score is not eligible for the MFC program. At Level II, a child requires nursing care and knowledge and more time and energy than would be spent on a foster child of the same age without medical or developmental problems. A child with this score is eligible for the MFC program. Children who score at Level III on the CCAT are those who require acute nursing care, extensive nursing knowledge and a great deal more time and energy than would be spent on a foster child of the same age without medical or developmental problems. These are children with complex health problems whose condition must be monitored by nurses with the assessment skills to make clinical judgments and to plan, carry out and evaluate nursing interventions. In the MFC model, children who scored at Level III were always placed in MFC homes with a registered nurse. On occasion, some children whose needs were scored at Level II were placed in MFC homes with licensed practical nurses with strong clinical backgrounds.

After processing is complete and placement decisions are made, a care plan is developed by the professional staff. A placement conference is held with the staff, the biologic parent(s) and the foster parents during which the final negotiations of the treatment plan takes place and placement details are finalized. The biologic parent meets the foster care case manager, the MFC foster parents, the clinical psychologist and other professional staff. All roles and responsibilities are reviewed with the parent and the ombudsman role of the psychologist is emphasized.

Each child placed in the MFC program has an individualized nursing care plan and a time-limited case management plan. In our model, the case plan requires participation by the biologic parents. The parent(s) of children placed in MFC must agree to the terms of the MFC placement and case plan; attend the preplacement meeting with the MFC foster parents and other professional staff and participate in scheduled home or clinic visits. The preplacement meeting enables the biologic parent(s) and the MFC foster parents to establish some sense of rapport and to begin discussion of treatment goals, roles and responsibilities, visitation schedules and performance agreements. A time is set for biologic parents to visit the MFC family in their home prior to a child's placement. This visit affords the biologic parents the opportunity to see where their child will be temporarily placed. Once the child is in care, however, a MFC family is given a "settling in" period of at least three days before biologic parents may visit. This delay gives the MFC parents the opportunity to get into a routine of nursing care without the additional intrusion of outsiders into their family system.

MFC families in our program were given a choice in the decision of whether to bring a specific child into their homes. Some nurses are expert in taking care of patients with burns; others feel comfortable with tracheotomies and apnea monitors. Some families are suited to parenting older children, while others prefer babies. Taking these variables into account tends to enhance the attachment of MFC foster families to children.

LEGAL ISSUES

Selection, approval and licensure of MFC homes must be carried out by an agency which already has legal authorization to do so. In our system, this is the state Department of Health and Rehabilitative Services. In other areas, it may be such agencies as Catholic Social Services or a similar agency. The official relationship between this program and an already established and accepted agency for licensure and monitoring is essential for risk management purposes. MFC homes are licensed by Health and Rehabilitative Services and meet all state licensing criteria. MFC families complete foster parent training, screening and evaluation that is required by other licensed foster families. In addition, the registered nurses in the program must maintain current licensure and certification in cardio-pulmonary resuscitation.

Respite care, alternative coverage, and baby-sitting quickly became issues that were addressed by coverage within the cadre of MFC parents and the use of a list of similarly qualified nurses approved by the licensing agency. In certain cases arrangements were made with local hospital providers to approve paid care for a few days of respite. This periodic relief is essential for the good mental health of the foster parents and their own biologic families.

Nurses who are licensed as MFC parents must have legal access to medical records and performance agreements as needed to facilitate goal accomplishment. In addition, they must have immediate access to the medical director to provide security and back-up in potential medical emergencies. Medical Foster Parents were incorporated into the professional staff of our program and hospital by being issued badges marked, "Registered Nurse" and "Medical Foster Care" (Foster & Whitworth, 1986).

To assure limitations of liability, Medical Foster Care parents can be contracted so as to be designated "agents of the state" and thus afforded sovereign immunity from civil prosecution. The nurse foster parents are also required to carry professional liability coverage.

RECRUITMENT

Recruitment of nurse foster parents is a joint endeavor of the MFC staff and the local district of Foster Care. Recruitment is an ongoing priority and takes a concentrated effort through advertisements in local newspapers and nursing publications. Presentations before professional nursing association meetings, community and church groups and surveying existing foster parents for those with nursing credentials may be efficacious. Once a program is operational, the best recruitment often takes place through word-of-mouth. Nurses who participate in the MFC program are generally those at home with school aged children, who wish to continue to practice nursing and add to their income but are not totally dependent on the earnings for basic living expenses.

COST/ANALYSIS

Since MFC is a marriage between classical foster care and a special system for assessment and tracking cases, each MFC family underwent a full licensure and certification process and was paid the current foster care rate applicable at the time of placement. In addition the monthly stipend was supplemented based on the acuity level determined by the CCAT. Payment for this supplement was provided by Children's Medical Services patient care funds. This state agency is responsible for providing care for medically complex or chronically ill children. The funds for program administration and staff were provided from the federal grant during the first three years and continued by a local hospital for children with chronic medical problems (Nemours Children's Hospital.) In the initial three years, comparative costs showed that the cost of five days of MFC was roughly equivalent to thirty days of hospital care. Initially, patient care payment ranged from three hundred dollars per month for a child whose score was at Level II on the CCAT to over a thousand dollars a month for a burned child with complex nursing care problems whose score was at Level III on the CCAT. In more recent years the costs of both hospital care and MFC have risen, but the rise in both has been proportionate and the ratio remains the same.

Restricting the program to participation of registered nurses is desirable but raises costs. If programs are carefully structured and adequate supervision is assured, a mix of registered nurses, licensed practical nurses and technicians with proven clinical skills can be effective.

CASE EXAMPLES

Two and a half year old Amy was hospitalized with scald burns inflicted by a relative. After two months of hospitalization, she went home to her parents who were overwhelmed with her care. The burns soon became infected and she returned to the hospital before being released into the temporary custody of a Medical Foster Family. She remained in MFC until her burns were healed and she then returned to her biological family (Foster, Davis, Whitworth & Skinner, 1982).

Missy at age seven was hospitalized and diagnosed as a failure-to-thrive child. She went home to her mother with multiple support services provided to the family. Six months later, she was admitted to the hospital for emergency surgery and a gastrostomy. Despite continued support services by a homemaker, a visiting nurse, and a protective service case manager, Missy was repeatedly hospitalized because of weight loss and neglect. She was placed in MFC until she gained enough weight to schedule reconstructive surgery of the esophagus. Upon her recovery, she returned to her biological family (Davis, Foster, & Whitworth, 1984).

Bobby, age three, suffered severe second and third degree scald burns inflicted by his mother. The maternal grandmother attempted to provide care after Bobby was released from the hospital, but his injuries became infected, requiring rehospitalization and grafting of the burn site. His burns healed and within six weeks he was playful and outgoing. The grandmother visited regularly in the MFC foster home and participated in his care. Her parenting improved as she relaxed her rigid, unrealistic expectations of a three year old. Bobby returned to his grandmother five months after placement in MFC.

Patty, a sixteen month old twin was hospitalized for nonorganic failure to thrive syndrome, severe depression and neglect. In the MFC home, she gained weight, and was soon walking, talking, and socializing appropriately. She and her siblings were later placed with relatives because of the mother's alcoholism.

OBSERVATIONS AND EVALUATION

To better understand the experiences of Medical Foster Families, interviews were held prior to acceptance and throughout the placement. Families described the phases they went through as they brought the children into their homes, nurtured them back to health and relinquished them to their parent(s), relatives or regular foster care placement.

When asked to describe their motives for participating in the MFC program, the nurses included the desire to continue the practice of nursing without the need to leave their own family and home. Some families said that the timing was right. Their own children were old enough to be somewhat independent, but young enough to play with a foster child. A pervasive motive for some MFC foster parents rested on strong religious convictions and the feeling that foster parenting is like a "mission." Others simply felt that they wanted to "give back" to society in some meaningful way and to share a nurturing family life with others less fortunate.

Despite their preparation through participation in foster parent training classes and planning conferences, MFC foster families often reacted with self doubts and feelings of isolation when a child was first placed in their homes. MFC families found that children upon release from a hospital environment into foster care went through stages of adjustment that could last for several days. Some families had not fully appreciated the twenty-four hour commitment of nursing responsibility.

Children who have been socialized to hospital life for much of their existence may behave in peculiar, unexpected ways. MFC foster families recognized both physical regression and psychosocial symptoms associated with long-term hospitalization. One child called every woman, "Mommie." Another forgot how to climb stairs and drew pictures of cars, airplanes and people the same size which was her perception from peering out a fifth floor hospital window. (Foster, Davis, Whitworth & Skinner, 1982).

As MFC families began to establish routines they experienced a sense of relief. Getting into routines is a theme that MFC families described within many levels of the experience. Routines took place in family relationships, nursing care of the medical foster child, and in dealing with the health care and social service systems. Nurse foster parents carried out prescribed nursing tasks and also made independent clinical nursing judgments, often conferring with the primary physician by telephone.

As children began to heal physically and emotionally and became a part of the MFC family system, the foster families delighted in their progress. Each foster child was incorporated into the MFC family system. Knowing that foster care is designed to provide temporary out of home placement, MFC families attempted to nurture and protect the biological family/child bond, but the effort seemed one-sided when biological families failed to call or visit. In an effort to motivate biological families to comply with performance agreements, external controls from the court, from the MFC case manager and from MFC families was sometimes indicated. Then as the children's physical status improved and biologic parents began to demonstrate appropriate behaviors, children were allowed to go home for brief visits. The visits produced a sense of ambivalence in the MFC families depending on the condition of the children when they returned.

At the point that MFC children are the happiest and healthiest and contributing to the foster family systems, plans must be made for their return to their biological families. MFC families worried about the physical and psychosocial needs of their foster children when they relinquished them to their biological families, and they wondered what kind of adjustment children would make in a less-than-optimal environment. In effect, MFC children become bicultural as a result of the experience. After spending months in the foster family setting, medical foster children speak with different grammar, use a different approach to problem solving and take on a different view of their world. For a time, these children are exposed to cultural advantages, effective parenting and unconditional love that may be in stark con-trast to what the future holds.

MFC families separated from the foster children in different ways. Some severed the relationship completely; some watched from a dis-tance—relying on reports from others; some made telephone calls at intervals; and one continued to maintain supportive relationship.

One MFC family whose foster child had been returned to the biologic family, articulated the family's meaning of the experience.

> We knew that we had taken a child who was hurting and had some measure of success with her inner healing, with her physical healing. She was well parented for the time period that she needed to go through.

> So having the feeling that we had done what we were called to do and had done what we had meant to do, all we could do was hope that it had given her a foundation that she could carry back into that family and function well with it.

Professionals working with MFC foster families have to know that the stages families go through in the process of the experience are important. As these foster parents work through the phases, they are going to having feelings of disquiet and uncertainty. An absolute necessity is that MFC foster families be helped to work through those stages with ample support and the least possible frustration. Anticipatory guidance can increase the awareness, visibility and structure of these stages and serves to expand coping strategies of MFC foster families.

The current nursing shortage has an effect on supply and recruitment of nurses for foster care. The MFC program has been replicated and expanded in the Tampa, Florida area.

REFERENCES

Davis, A. B., Foster, P. H., & Whitworth, J. M. (1984). Medical foster family care: A cost-effective solution to a community problem. *Child Welfare 63*(4), 341–349.

Foster, P. H., Davis, A. B., Whitworth, J. M. & Skinner, R. G. (1982) Medical foster care: An alternative nursing practice. *American Journal of Maternal Child Nursing. 7*(4), 245–248.

Foster, P. H. & Whitworth, J. M. (1986). Medical foster care: An alternative to long-term hospitalization. *Children Today 14*(4), 12–16.

Gurdin, P. & Anderson, G. R. (1987). Quality care for ill children: AIDS-specialized foster family homes. *Child Welfare. 66*(4), 291–302.

Karniski, W., Van Buren, L. & Cupoli, J. M. (1986). A treatment program for failure to thrive: A cost/effectiveness analysis. *Child Abuse Neglect. 10*(4), 471–478.

Shah, C. P. & Poulos, S. (1974). Assessing needs and board rates for handicapped children in foster family care. Progress report. *Child Welfare 53*(1), 31–37.

Tourse, P. & Gundersen, L. (May–June 1988) Fostering children with AIDS: Policies in progress. *Children Today.* pp. 15–19.

Whitworth, J. M., Lanier, M. W., Skinner, R. G. & Lund, N. L. (1981) A multidisciplinary hospital based team for child abuse cases. *Child Welfare 60*(2), 233–243.

CHAPTER 11

PRESCRIBED PEDIATRIC EXTENDED CARE: THE FAMILY CENTERED HEALTH CARE ALTERNATIVE FOR MEDICALLY AND TECHNOLOGY DEPENDENT CHILDREN

PATRICIA M. PIERCE
DONNA G. LESTER
DEBORAH E. FRAZE

INTRODUCTION

The health care needs for some children have changed dramatically in recent years. Just a decade ago, the survival rate for children born extremely prematurely, with very complex syndromes, or with life threatening congenital anomalies was small enough to escape widespread attention. Most of these children died at birth or shortly thereafter. Furthermore, for the few remaining survivors, the family home was almost always able to incorporate the child with special health care needs into the family structure.

Now, however, available medical technology rescues many children and supplements or replaces the child's inadequate physiological development with technological and/or mechanical interventions that enable the child to survive and grow. Often these artificial supports can be discontinued as the child matures physiologically. But, in the interim, highly skilled personnel and specialized settings are often necessary to monitor, assess, and regulate the technological support systems.

Up to now, few care alternatives were available to the families of these medically and technology dependent children. The parents could 1) leave the child in the hospital for extended periods of time, 2) hire nurses to provide care in the home, or 3) one parent could remain at home to care for the child. If the parents left the child in the hospital setting, the costs associated with hospital care could exhaust insurance policy benefits within the first few months of the child's life. If private duty nurses were employed to provide care in the home, the result was expensive, sometimes disruptive to the family, and restricted the child to an environment void of peers and frequently limited in developmentally appropriate experiences. For families that needed two incomes to maintain financial stability or for single parents, the choice frequently was to leave the medically dependent child at the hospital or occasionally to assign custody to a state agency.

WHAT IS PRESCRIBED PEDIATRIC EXTENDED CARE (PPEC)?

The Prescribed Pediatric Extended Care (PPEC) Center is a non-residential, family-centered health care service prescribed by a physician for children who are medically and/or technologically dependent. As part of the continuum of care for medically dependent children, the PPEC center provides a triad of necessary services: day medical care, developmental programming, and parental training. The PPEC Center provides a less restrictive alternative to hospitalization and reduces the isolation often experienced by the home-bound, medically dependent child.

The PPEC Center is a cost-effective, medically safe setting for medically fragile children who require sophisticated medical treatments for extended periods of time. Only those children who require skilled medical and nursing interventions, such as, mechanical ventilation, parenteral (intravenous) nutrition, intravenous fluids/medications, oxygen therapy, breathing treatments, tracheostomy care, enteral feedings, etc. are eligible for PPEC services. Highly skilled pediatric registered nurses provide expert nursing care; licensed physical, occupational, and oral-motor therapists are available on site to provide prescribed therapies for children attending a PPEC, Inc. Center.

This community-based health care delivery alternative represents an innovative, cost effective approach to address the complex service needs of children who require sophisticated technological interventions and, at the same time, provides a home-like environment that fosters growth and development. The PPEC Center offers a less restrictive alternative to hospitalization and reduces the isolation of home-bound care. The staff of the PPEC Center uses a family-centered approach to provide the triad of necessary services: day medical care, developmental planning and intervention, and parent training.

A major premise of the comprehensive program offered at the PPEC Center is that the quality of life of the child and family can be significantly enhanced by maintaining a family-centered focus and addressing all of the complex health, psychosocial, and training needs. The PPEC Center program encourages families to participate with the health care professionals as an equal partner in their child's care and, through participation, gain the understanding and confidence necessary to fully integrate their medically fragile child into family life.

WHY IS THE PPEC NEEDED?

The children receiving PPEC services require sophisticated technological interventions until they are more mature physiologically. For these children, the PPEC Center serves as a transitional health care setting that can support them until they are healthy enough to enter regular, mainstream child care facilities. Children admitted to the PPEC Center may require mechanical ventilation, hyperalimentation, oxygen, apnea monitoring, or have a variety of congenital anomalies, severe chronic illnesses, and genetic syndromes that require extended and unusual interventions. All require highly skilled professional nursing services. Prior to admission to the PPEC Center, the child's physician completes a written medical treatment plan and the physician receives regular updates regarding the child's progress and changes in the child's condition.

The population of children who are medically and/or technology dependent is steadily increasing. These children must "use a medical technology to compensate for the loss of normal use of a vital body function, and require substantial daily skilled nursing care to avert death or further disability" (U.S. Congress, Office of Technology Assessment [OTA], 1987). For the most part, medically dependent children are born very prematurely, or have an acute or chronic, complex health impairment that requires unusual and extended treatment.

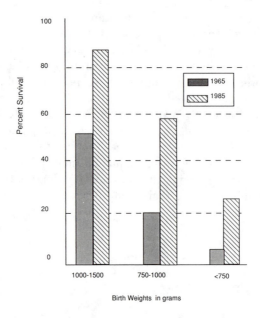

Figure 11.1. Survival Rates for Very Low Birth Weight Infants.

Premature Infants

In Florida alone more than 4,000 children annually are born prematurely and are treated in one of twelve regional perinatal centers. Several hundred more premature infants receive neonatal intensive care in community hospitals throughout the state. As is illustrated in Figure 11.1, care provided through these units has resulted in dramatic increases in the survival rates of very low birth weight infants (Lyon, 1985).

Although most of these very small infants ultimately develop and grow normally, many require an extraordinary amount of medical support, (e.g., ventilator assistance, apnea monitoring, supplemental oxygen), for months or years. For example, national estimates indicate that broncho-pulmonary dysplasia, a leading cause of respiratory problems, occurs in approximately 9,000 infants per year (U.S. Congress OTA, 1987). Because of their dependence on technological support, many of these children remain hospitalized even after they are medically stable enough to be discharged from the intensive care hospital setting.

**Table 11.1. Summary of Conditions, Services and Diagnoses of Children
who are Candidates for PPEC, Inc. Centers.**

Condition	Services	Diagnoses
Acute and/or chronic medical or surgical condition conditions cystic	IV medications and therapy, suctioning, complex alimentation	Severe infection, postoperative myopathies, severe fibrosis, malabsorption and short gut syndromes
Chronic respiratory condition tracheomalacia	Mechanical ventilation, cardiopulmonary monitoring, tracheostomy care	Chronic BPD, Post CNS infection, progressive CNS disease
Terminal conditions	Dialysis, chemotherapy, oxygen	Renal disease, cancer

Children with Complex Health Care Needs

In addition to those children experiencing the sequelae of prematurity, significant numbers of children have complex medical conditions and require extensive and sophisticated technological support. For example, nationally, approximately 45,000 children require monitoring for apnea, 3,000 are dependent on external respiratory support, and 8,275 receive extended intravenous therapy either for hyperalimentation or medications (U.S. Congress OTA, 1987). Table 11.1 provides an abbreviated summary of types of children who could require the extensive therapeutic services available in a PPEC Center.

The exact number of children with complex conditions is difficult to discern. Extensive analyses indicate that approximately 10 percent of all children have a chronic condition, and of these, about 1 percent have disease manifestations which require the kind of services available in a PPEC Center (Hobbs and Perrin, 1985; Hughes, Johnson, Simons, Rosenbaum, 1986; U.S. Congress OTA, 1987). Based on these incidence estimates, there are approximately 2,500 infants and children in Florida alone who would be appropriate for and benefit from PPEC Center services. Furthermore, health care industry experts clearly recognize, and predict, that the next 10 years will bring a marked increase in the number and use of cost effective alternatives to extended inpatient hospital care (Arthur A. Anderson & Company and American College of Hospital Administrators, 1984; Hughes, Johnson, Simons & Rosenbaum, 1986; Lopez, 1987; U.S. Congress OTA, 1987).

LAYING THE GROUNDWORK FOR A QUALITY PROGRAM

National Model Standards

A key step in the development and implementation of the PPEC Center was the establishment of Model Standards to guide and evaluate this new health care delivery alternative. The model standards were developed in association with a panel of recognized experts in the fields of child health and child development. Subspecialist pediatricians were included in order to assure that the physiological needs of medically fragile children would be addressed adequately and appropriately. Specialized expertise regarding the pyscho-social/developmental needs of medically fragile children was provided by panel members with backgrounds in pediatric nursing, child psychology, and developmental pediatrics. Public program officials from Title V and Medicaid provided guidance concerning existing regulations and financial aspects applicable to pediatric care programs. The parent of a medically complex child served as a parent/consumer consultant to the panel. Panel members adopted the philosophy that the standards would contain criteria they would expect if they had a medically fragile child who was going to receive services in the PPEC Center.

The standards define admission requirements and procedures, staffing ratios and staff qualifications, program components, quality assurance requirements, building requirements, and emergency procedures. The quality assurance (QA) program in the standards provides a comprehensive method for evaluating the entire PPEC Center program. In addition to the PPEC's internal QA procedure, the State of Florida Office of Licensure and Certification is responsible for a yearly, on-site inspection of each center. Health care professionals are included on the state inspection team. Further, because some of the children receiving PPEC services are funded by state general revenue, professionals from the state Program for Children with Special Needs (formerly Crippled Children's Program) conduct an on-site program review of services.

The standards were tested in the prototype PPEC Center in Tampa, FL. The thoughtful, hard work of the expert panel resulted in a set of standards that have needed minimal adjustments during the last four years.

Licensing PPEC Centers in Florida

An important part of the PPEC Center project was to establish separate licensure category to assure that all such centers would have to conform to the child and family oriented guidelines included in the standards. In 1987 the Florida legislature passed the law licensing PPEC Centers, thereby establishing a legal mechanism for certifying the quality of care provided to medically fragile children in the state. The Florida law has since been passed by at least two additional states—Delaware and Kentucky. The PPEC standards formed the basis for the administrative rules to implement the licensure process.

Passage of legislation in Florida has contributed to PPEC's acceptance by the health care providers and payers. With the enactment of this legislation, which assures minimum service standards and quality assurance requirements, insurance companies are able to reimburse PPEC Center services. Further, the language of the law demands that the PPEC Center program be comprehensive and family-centered.

THE PPEC CENTER PROGRAM

The PPEC Center program combines extensive pediatric specialty nursing care with individual and group developmental activities. Some of the children at the PPEC Center receive a combination of PPEC services during the day and in-home nursing at night. Only these children who require skilled medical and nursing interventions, such as, mechanical ventilation, parenteral (intravenous) nutrition, intravenous fluids/medications, oxygen therapy, breathing treatments, tracheostomy care, enteral feedings, etc. are eligible for PPEC services. Admission to a PPEC Center must be prescribed by the child's physician. Highly skilled pediatric registered nurses provide expert nursing care; licensed physical, occupational, and oral-motor therapists are available on site to provide prescribed therapies for children attending a PPEC Center. As the family becomes more comfortable and confident in caring for their medically fragile child, in-home services can be reduced and finally discontinued. Thus, the PPEC Center serves as a transitional setting that can support medically fragile children until they are healthy enough to enter mainstream child care facilities.

The PPEC Center program involves development and implementation of a comprehensive Protocol of Care following a physician's prescription for admission. Included in the protocol are measurable outcome objectives for the child's medical needs, developmental achievement, and parent competence/confidence for caring for the child in the home. In addition to guiding the child's PPEC program of care, the measurable outcome objectives assist the professionals and family to determine when the child is ready for discharge from the PPEC Center.

The staff of the PPEC Center assume their role as a part of the entire continuum of care for the children. One of the nursing staff serves as the case management nurse for a child prior to and after admission to the PPEC Center. This case manager nurse and the PPEC Center Managing Director (also a pediatric specialty nurse) work with the hospital staff, family, and insurance carrier to facilitate the timely and orderly hospital discharge and PPEC admission. They include individuals from the hospital's multi-disciplinary team as well as the child's parent(s)/guardian(s) in the development of the comprehensive PPEC Protocol of Care. Further, each PPEC Center has a designated coordinator who serves as the liaison among the PPEC Center, the child and family, and the provider community—including health care, education, economic services, social support services, and supply/equipment vendors. Interfacing with the other services involved with the child and providing ongoing case management offer the best methods for maintaining continuity of care and reducing the chance of costly, fragmentation of service delivery.

When the child and family arrive at the PPEC Center each morning, a member of the registered nursing staff examines the child to ascertain his/her current health status and to assure that he/she is free of contagious diseases. The nurses and family members also use this time to discuss how the child has been overnight and whether there have been any new developments in the child's response to the medical plan of care.

The atmosphere of the PPEC Center is family-centered and parent training in both technical skills and anticipatory guidance receives special emphasis. Experience has clearly demonstrated that parents who feel confident about their ability to manage their child's medical needs are more astute consumers of health care resources. Further, the parents have identified the PPEC Center as a place where they can participate in normal parenting events, such as having a picture of their child on Santa's knee or celebrating birthdays with peers. Parents of children receiving PPEC services can assume a more normal life style and maintain or return to employment knowing their child is receiving expert and loving care. In fact, families whose children have received PPEC Center services are extremely enthusiastic about the program and repeatedly suggest that the concept be expanded, "so other parents and children have the advantage of PPEC Center services."

An outstanding feature of the PPEC Center concept has been its broad acceptance. Physicians enthusiastically prescribe the PPEC Center for their medically dependent patients because the Center provides the comprehensive array of services that children with complex illnesses require. Furthermore, the physicians rely on receiving regular and accurate information about their patients' medical status. They have more opportunities to "fine tune" the treatment plan, thereby reducing the number of times a child might experience an avoidable exacerbation of his or her illness.

The children benefit greatly from being in the PPEC Center. The nursing staff are experts in the care of children with conditions requiring sophisticated therapies, and also are trained to incorporate developmental stimulation into the child's routine daily treatment schedule. Children receive needed speech, occupational, and physical therapies from pediatric experts who, because they all provide therapy at the PPEC Center, have the opportunity to freely consult with each other regarding the child's progress. The result is that the overall developmental progress of the children is enhanced.

The PPEC Center receives referrals from a variety of providers, payers, and consumers. Most often the child's physician will make a direct referral for PPEC services for one of his/her patients. Many times, however, insurance company representatives and case managers from payers and third party administrators make referrals to the PPEC Center. Sometimes parents have learned about the PPEC Center and inquire about how they can have their child admitted.

REIMBURSEMENT FOR PPEC CENTER SERVICES

Establishing a Fee Structure

Charges for PPEC Center services were originally based on hourly rates. However, at the urging of insurance claims specialists, the pricing structure was converted to a per diem rate. The per diem rate for a child is established by 1) assigning an acuity level for the child's medical condition, 2) determining the number and kind of additional prescribed therapeutic services, 3) calculating the amount of supplies required, and 4) charging a predetermined portion of the retainer for the pediatrician who serves as the PPEC Center Medical Director.

Five acuity levels have been defined and range from respite care to the one-on-one care that is required by a child receiving mechanical ventilation. The cost of ancillary services, (i.e., speech, physical, and occupational therapy), are based on charges for the therapists' time.

Health insurers have been very receptive to the PPEC Center concept. Many of the major insurers (e.g., Humana, Aetna, Metropolitan, Prudential, Travelers) have not only reimbursed PPEC claims, but also have facilitated the claims process by assigning a specific individual to assist with PPEC Center claims. PPEC, Inc. is a preferred provider for Humana and in process of establishing a similar arrangement with Blue Cross, Health Options, and CHAMPUS. Unique procedure codes for PPEC services have been developed to facilitate and expedite processing of claims. Further, many insurers have indicated an interest in the expansion of the PPEC Center system to other locations in Florida and nationally.

Children's Medical Services (CMS), Florida's program for children with special health care needs, has also exhibited a very positive response to PPEC services. PPEC, Inc. has a rate agreement contract for services at both the Tampa and Miami PPEC, Inc. Centers. Because CMS can extend its patient service dollars to provide appropriate services to greater numbers of children, program officials have expressed a willingness to establish similar reimbursement rate agreements for PPEC services in other locations in Florida.

Public officials in Florida are also exploring mechanisms for using Medicaid dollars as a source of reimbursement for PPEC, Inc. services. Because of the current cap on Medicaid reimbursable hospital days in Florida, there has been little incentive for Medicaid to consider alternative care delivery systems for children who are medically fragile. Florida officials are in the process of increasing the number of Medicaid hospital days, which should result in defining a mechanism for establishing a state match for Medicaid reimbursement.

Figure 11.2 compares the per diem costs for PPEC Center services with hospital and in-home nursing. From this graph, it is easy to see why insurers are willing, and even anxious, to reimburse PPEC Center services.

Upon close examination, PPEC's cost advantage is even more dramatic. Table 11.2 below compares the services included in the per diem rate for hospitals, home nursing and PPEC Centers.

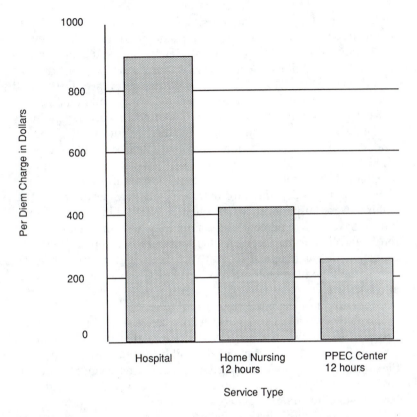

Figure 11.2. Daily Cost Comparison Among Alternatives.

Table 11.2. Services Included in Per Diem Rate.

Hospital	Home Nursing	PPEC, Inc. Center
Nursing Care	Nursing Care	Nursing Care
Child Life Worker		Developmentalist
Social Worker		Occupational Therapy
		Physical Therapy
		Speech Therapy
		Case Management

RECOGNITION AND GROWTH OF THE PPEC CENTER CONCEPT

A Cost Effectiveness Evaluation

An evaluation of the PPEC Center was conducted by independent evaluators to determine whether significant differences existed with regard to costs, functional status, morbidity and mortality between children cared for at the PPEC Center and a matched control group cared for by traditional means. Results of this study support the cost effectiveness of the PPEC Center. Significant differences were found when the health care expenditures of families with children receiving PPEC Center services were compared with health care expenditures of families whose children either remained in the hospital for extended stays or received in-home nursing (Kilpatrick, Miller, Clarke, 1988).

Although hospital re-admission data were insufficient for critical analysis of morbidity, the information seemed to indicate that PPEC children were hospitalized less frequently than children in the control group. Seventy-five percent of the families whose children were currently enrolled or had been enrolled in the PPEC Center reported a reduction in unanticipated health care visits and health care costs during the time their children received PPEC services (Kilpatrick, et al., 1988).

Other findings included dramatic differences in the stress level reported by families. The families were asked a series of 25 questions designed to assess the life stress 1) prior to the time of the child's birth or injury, 2) at the time of the child's birth or injury, and 3) at the time of the interview, in order to determine changes in family stress levels. Some of the questions included were: "Do (did) you have enough free time?", "Do (did) you have enough privacy?", "Do (did) you have enough time for each other?", "Do (did) you get enough sleep?" "Do (did) you have enough money to do the things you want to do?" Although control group and PPEC families reported similar increases in stress at the time of diagnosis, the stress level for the control group remained significantly higher. PPEC families reported stress levels almost comparable to what would be expected for families without a medically or technology dependent child.

Recognition of PPEC

National acceptance and support for the PPEC Center concept was confirmed when the PPEC Center in Tampa received the 1988 Award for Innovation from the Association for the Care of Children's Health (ACCH). ACCH is an international, multidisciplinary organization and the award from ACCH represents a seal of approval from providers, insurers, and consumers.

The PPEC Center concept was recommended as "an innovative alternative in the continuum of care" by the Congressional Task Force on Technology Dependent Children (1988). The Task Force acknowledged the need for day health facilities for severely compromised infants and indicated that PPEC expedites the development of such programs within Florida and could serve as a model for other states.

SUMMARY

The advent of the PPEC Center represents an important link in the continuum of care for children who are medically and/or technology dependent. The growing interest in containing health care costs coupled with the need to provide a comprehensive, developmentally appropriate environment for children with complex health impairments strongly suggests that the PPEC model will be widely replicated. By providing comprehensive and coordinated medical, developmental and parent training services, the PPEC Center facilitates the child and family's progress toward optimal functioning in a cost effective manner.

REFERENCES

Arthur A. Anderson & Co. and American College of Hospital Administrators, (1984). Health Trends for the 1990s. Report of the Delphi Study, Dallas: Author.

Congressional Task Force on Technology Dependent Children. (1988). Fostering Home and Community-Based Care for Technology-Dependent Children. Report of the Task Force on Technology-Dependent Children. (HCFA Pub. No. 88-02171). Washington, D.C.: U.S. Government Printing Office.

Hobbs, H., Perrin, J. M. (1985). *Issues in the Care of Children with Chronic Illness*. San Francisco: Jossey-Bass Publishers.

Hughes, F., Johnson, K., Simons, J., & Rosenbaum, S. (1986). *Maternal and Child Health Data Book*. Washington, D.C.: Children's Defense Fund.

Kilpatrick, K., Miller, M., Clarke, L. (1988). An evaluation of the relative economic and psychological stress on families of children enrolled in the prescribed pediatric extended care center and those of children cared for in other settings, February 1988. In P. M. Pierce & S. A. Freedman, *Final Report Prescribed Pediatric Extended Care: Medical Day Care A Cost Effective Alternative for Families of Medically Dependent Children* (HHS Grant MCJ-123490) Gainesville, FL: Family Health and Habilitative Services, Inc.

Lopez, L. (1987). High cost illness among children: A sleeping giant, *Business and Health.* *13*(4), 16–19.

Lyon, J. (1985). *Playing God in the nursery.* New York: W.W. Norton & Company.

U.S. Congress, Office of Technology Assessment. (1987). Technology-Dependent Children: Hospital vs. Home Care—A Technical Memorandum. (OTA-TM-H-38). Washington, D.C.: U. S. Government Printing Office.

CHAPTER 12

THE HEALTH CARE-CHILD WELFARE PARTNERSHIP: THE TRANSITION OF MEDICALLY COMPLEX CHILDREN TO THE COMMUNITY*

NEIL J. HOCHSTADT
DIANE M. YOST

INTRODUCTION

Throughout the country there is a growing number of children residing in hospitals who are seriously chronically ill with complex medical conditions and/or complex home health care needs (Office of Technology Assessment, 1987). Others have used the term medically fragile or technologically dependent to describe this population. It is generally agreed that many medically complex children would be best served in home care environments. Currently, few programs exist for developing and maintaining this population of children outside of medical institutions. As a result, they may remain hospitalized for months and often years.

Limited information suggests that the number of medically complex children requiring long-term care is increasing (Newacheck, Budetti & McManus, 1984; Office of Technology Assessment, 1987). It is estimated that ten percent of all chronically ill children are medically

*Reprinted with permission from article published in 1989, volume 18, number 1, *Children's Health Care*, The Journal of the Association for the Care of Children's Health (ACCH), and reprinted with permission from ACCH. ACCH is a multidisciplinary organization whose mission is to ensure that all aspects of children's health care are family-centered, psychosocially sound, and developmentally appropriate. For further information about membership or other resources contact: ACCH, 7910 Woodmont Avenue, Suite 300, Bethesda, MD 20814
This project was supported in part by the Department of Health and Human Services, Office of Human Development Services, Administration for Children, Youth and Families, under grant 90-CW-0790.

or technologically dependent (Hobbs, Perrin & Ireys, 1985). Further it is estimated that there are up to 17,000 children requiring ventilator assistance, parenteral nutrition, prolonged use of intravenous drugs and other device-based respiratory or nutritional support. If children requiring apnea monitoring, renal dialysis, and device-associated nursing care are included, this number may increase by 80,000 (Office of Technology Assessment, 1987). The actual number of chronically health impaired children residing in acute care hospitals on an on-going basis is unknown. However, a review of children hospitalized in Minneapolis-St. Paul revealed that 624 patients, representing 31,500 days of inpatient care, did not require hospitalization in acute care hospitals (Bieter, Kasbohm, Kaufman & Aufderheide, 1981). This study estimated that there would be a continuing need for 45 pediatric transitional care beds in the Minneapolis-St. Paul metropolitan area.

A variety of factors have conspired to place a greater emphasis on home care for medically complex children. These factors include the following: (1) the increasing number of children with a variety of chronic diseases (Gortmaker, 1985); (2) the increasing survival rate of seriously impaired neonates due to improved medical care and technology (Kohrman, 1985); (3) changes in public policy such as Public Law 94-142 (Education of the Handicapped Act, 1970) and Public Law 96-272 (Social Security Act, 1935) emphasizing the care of children in the "least restrictive environment," as well as other legislation for developmentally and physically disabled individuals. Recent changes in medical economics, reflected in such developments as diagnosis related groups (DRG'S) have also made home care a greater imperative for this population of children.

Merkens (1983) identified several groups of medically complex children who can be considered for home care: (1) children who, while generally medically stable, have high technological needs for therapies, treatments, equipment, continuous observation, monitoring (e.g., children with long-term tracheostomies, feeding gastrostomies, intermittent or continuous ventilator support, children requiring total parenteral nutrition); (2) children hospitalized for a change in medical management or counseling for adaptation (e.g., the out of control diabetic or asthmatic child who can no longer be managed effectively by his/her parents); (3) children recuperating from complicated surgery or accidents whose illness involves a prolonged recovery during which time skilled nursing and/or medical care is required; (4) children "in transition" from tertiary centers to home care (e.g. children who are generally medically stable but their parents or caregivers require a setting in which to learn the technical and developmental aspects of their care management); (5) children who are medically stable but for whom there is no satisfactory home setting.

Among these children there is a small but growing number who have been hospitalized in acute care hospitals because alternative homecare is unavailable. These children receive a higher level of medical and nursing care than they require at unnecessarily high costs. They also experience the detrimental effects of long-term care in acute hospital settings unable to support their developmental needs or the psychosocial needs of their families. The cost of caring for these children in acute care hospitals is high and is generally supported by public funding agencies such as Medicaid, State Departments of Public Aid or State Services for Crippled Children. The Office of Technology Assessment (1987) notes that for ventilator dependent children in Illinois, medicaid payments for the last month of hospitalization averages $16,948, while monthly home care payments averaged $6,358. For the same population having some private insurance coverage, the cost of the last month of hospital care averaged $26,616 while similar home care averaged $6,922. Similar savings were noted in Maryland and Louisiana. However, this is such a new population of children, with diverse medical conditions and home health care needs, that more research is needed to assess the relative cost effectiveness of home care. It is clear that the cost to these children in terms of compromised development, lost educational opportunities, and arrested emotional growth, as a result of growing up in a hospital environment, is incalculable (Dombro & Haas, 1970; Tekely & Dittemore, 1978; Vernon, Schulman & Foley, 1966).

AN INNOVATIVE RESPONSE TO A GROWING PROBLEM

The need to develop alternative models of community based care for this population is readily apparent. These children represent a significant challenge to health care and child welfare providers. The challenge resides not in their technical or medical management, but in the professional community's ability to develop alternative community based services to appropriately meet their needs.

The federally supported Medical Foster Parent Program (MFPP) reported on here (Department of Health and Human Services, 1986) is a unique program to develop home care resources for a significant sub-population of medically complex children—those medically complex children residing in hospitals for whom a return to their biological parents is not possible. This two year project was designed to determine if collaboration between a pediatric hospital and a child welfare agency could develop the requisite community resources to transition medically complex children from the hospital to a home care setting. La Rabida Children's Hospital and Research Center (LRCH) is the pediatric chronic disease hospital of the University of Chicago. The hospital and its outpatient programs care for children with a wide range of chronic illnesses and handicapping conditions. Children's Home and Aid Society (CHASI) is a state-wide, non-profit, private child welfare agency providing a wide range of child placement services, child and family counseling, research and professional training.

There have been several attempts to develop community based family care for the growing number of medically complex children. Project Impact (1984) developed a partnership with the Developmental Evaluation Clinic at Children's Hospital (Boston) to work more closely with developmentally delayed and special needs children to increase permanency planning through adoption. The Medical Foster Care Family Project, (Davis, Foster, & Whitworth, 1984) established in Florida by the Children's Medical Service Program, developed a program of foster care using registered nurses who became licensed foster parents. The Baby House (United Cerebral Palsy Association, 1986) also located in Florida, provides small cottage living with trained staff for medically complex and developmentally delayed children. The Prescribed Pediatric Extended Care Center (Pierce, Freedman & Reese, 1987) is a non-residential, family-centered, outpatient health care service in Florida, providing day medical care, developmental programing, and parental training for medically complex children. A more extensive description of some of these programs can be found in this section.

The MFPP and those programs mentioned above are viewed as a logical extension of the current multidisciplinary model of health care. As patients' needs and health care services become more specialized, higher levels of coordination and collaboration have become essential. The placement of children outside the hospital, with substitute care providers, demands the extension of the multidisciplinary team to include a range of community services (e.g., health care, child welfare, social service and funding).

The MFPP was designed to provide comprehensive medical foster care to sixteen children requiring high levels of nursing care, technologic support, and extensive involvement of caretakers in their medical management. Unlike the project described by Davis, Foster and Whitworth (1984), the MFPP did not specifically recruit professional nurses (R.N.'s). Children in this project are currently under the custody or guardianship of the Illinois Department of Children and Family Services. While they are medically ready for discharge, their parents are unable or unwilling to provide home care. The project requires the integration of child welfare expertise (e.g., foster family recruitment, development and placement) with health care expertise (e.g., medical management and training in home health care and follow-up). The core components of the program include specialized foster family recruitment, training foster parents in the medical, developmental and psychosocial care of medically complex children, placement of children in suitable foster families, and provision of on-going support and follow-up services.

To date eleven children have been referred to the MFPP for transitioning to community care. Project children present with conditions of broncopulmonary dysplasia, Pierre Robin Syndrome, quadriplegia, central hypoventilation syndrome, ventilator dependency, and dependency on phrenic pacers. Many have developmental delays, all have complex treatment regimines (e.g., frequent medications, nebulization treatments, and suctioning at periodic intervals, etc.). In one case the disability resulted from physical abuse. This circumstance generated a great deal of stress for the health care and child welfare professionals. To date, six of the children have been transitioned into homes within the community. Five of these have been placed with foster families and one with relatives. Of the five remaining children, a potential foster family has been identified for one with birth parent reunification identified for another three children currently have no community resources identified.

Foster families have been recruited from the general population and the existing pool of licensed foster families. The recruitment of these families has been accomplished through the development of a special program utilizing media, advertisements, videotapes and community presentations. The expertise of both LRCH and CHASI is essential to provide families with the skills they need to manage children with special needs at home. Simultaneously, prospective foster parents participated in an eight session training program in the care of medically complex children. The eight session training curriculum covers the following areas of foster care for medically complex children: foster parents as part of the health care team, medical and nursing care, emotional factors in the care of medically complex children, understanding the foster care system, separation and loss, behavioral management of foster children, and community resources. They also participated in a foster home assessment and licensing study (approximately 6–12 interviews) to assure that state licensing standards were met. Additional child specific medical training precedes placement within the home.

One of the most important accomplishments of the MFPP has been the identification of problems and barriers to community placement of medically complex children. Below are presented our findings regarding the challenges facing those involved in transitioning medically complex children to the community.

THE CHALLENGE FOR COMMUNITY BASED SERVICE PROVIDERS

This is a new population of children for most community service providers. In order to effectively serve this population, community service agencies (e.g., social service and child welfare agencies, home health care agencies, schools, vendors, funding agencies) must learn new skills such as medical terminology, medical management, sharing roles, and developing cooperative relationships with a myriad of new co-collaborators.

Typically community agencies have clear-cut rules and categorical definitions for their services. There are few rules currently available surrounding the care of medically complex children in the community. For example, school districts have little experience educating ventilator dependent children. Few ground rules exist for funding, curriculum, classroom placement or whether these children should be in a school setting at all. School personnel, parents, health care personnel, home health agencies, funding agencies and others must negotiate new rules and relationships if these children are to be educated in a community setting.

> A local suburban school system was responsible for providing schooling for B.A., who has a tracheostomy. The school, which did not have a nurse on staff adamantly refused to provide one and challenged the family to take legal action. This situation was finally resolved after much advocacy at the local and state level but only after B.A. lost one year of formal schooling.

Role diffusion is most clearly seen in the interface between home health care personnel and family members. The intrusion of home health care personnel into family life (e.g., 24 hours of nursing care, 7 days per week) often causes great stress on the family and on health care providers (Moos & Tsu, 1977). Stress results from the struggle to redefine roles of both family members and health care providers vis-a-vis the care of the child.

A.S.'s foster family was upset because the nurses disciplined him in ways inconsistent with the family value system. Further, one nurse began to carry him around all day rather than encouraging him to walk.

J.H.'s nurse encouraged him to call her "mommy" when his foster mother was not present and talked about adopting the child herself.

The family must attempt to incorporate multiple care-givers into their family system (e.g., three shifts of nursing per day, physical therapists, vendors, etc.) while health care providers must develop strategies for providing services in an unfamiliar environment (i.e., the home). Often this struggle is not recognized as a role or boundary problem but is played out as a control struggle. The family perceives that they know what is best for the child and can modify or change the health care regimen as they see fit; the home health care providers perceive that they are the health care professionals and know what is best for the child. Similarly, service providers who typically do not interface with each other may be obliged to redefine roles and boundaries as they work to provide home care for these children. For example, child welfare agencies typically make all decisions regarding recruitment and placement of foster children; hospital personnel have little or no experience in this area. In the project reported on in this paper the child welfare agency involved, CHASI, and the pediatric hospital, LRCH, had to redefine their roles to share this responsibility. Learning to share roles, redefine boundaries and develop trusting relationships are crucial milestones in developing the ability to transition children to community care.

THE CHALLENGE FOR HEALTH CARE PROVIDERS

To effectively transition medically complex children to the community, the hospital based multidisciplinary team must redefine its role, and the role of its members, and broaden the definition of the team. Since many medically complex children are relatively stable, the extra-medical aspects of their care may take precedence creating an unsettling effect on the homeostasis of the medical team. For example, non-medical issues such as discharge planning, training parents, acquisition of funds, and linking with community agencies may take priority over medical issues. Extending the traditional hospital based health care team to embrace the requisite community agencies and family members is crucial to caring for medically complex children. Since these children require very complex home health care plans, discharge planning is extraordinarily difficult and time consuming. It has been our experience that lengthy delays by funding agencies, complex training of families, negotiations with various community agencies, medical exigencies, and bureaucratic delays tax the morale of the most experienced staff.

Lastly, health care teams face the challenge of developing effective working relationships with hospital administrators. These children often require lengthy hospital stays causing a great deal of apprehension amongst cost conscious administrators. It is essential for the health care team to educate hospital administrators to the difficulties and complexities of discharge planning for this population of children. It is helpful to provide hospital administrators with detailed accounts of how labor intensive discharge planning is, of the ongoing efforts to effect discharge plans, and with routine updates as to the status of discharge planning for each child.

THE CHALLENGE FOR FAMILIES

The nature of foster care demands that the lives of foster families and birth families be intertwined with a view toward the best interests of the child and a determination of the long term placement arrangements. During this process both sets of families are beset by strong feelings and challenges as a result of the placement arrangement which require agency intervention and support.

The birth parents experience profound feelings of separation and loss when their child, who is not a perfect child, spends large periods of time or perhaps all of their early lives in the hospital. The impact on their self esteem, which for many may already be low, can be devastating. The event of foster placement of the medically complex child may be seen as one more failure for some birth families. Or, it may be the event that permits them to more adequately parent their healthy children.

The foster families also experience difficulties with issues of separation and loss. They may constantly face the fear that their foster child, with whom they have formed profound attachments, will be lost to them when returned home. Their fears may be heightened if the birth family situation is perceived as marginal or potentially injurious. However, while the child is in their home they experience some powerful challenges in carrying out their fostering function.

Typically, foster families struggle with defining their varied and complex roles. There are many demands upon them to function as though the children truly belonged to them. They are the ones who provide the day to day nurture and support while performing the difficult tasks associated with the care of medically complex children. Additionally, they must negotiate a vast array of other systems, including nursing, technologic supports, funding and social services. The vast intrusions which the systems produce can be overwhelming for even the most highly functioning families.

> J.H.'s foster family called approximately 100 pediatricians before they found one both familiar with tracheostomy patients and willing to accept the medicaid card.

It becomes the responsibility of the health care and social service professionals to provide assistance with the myriad issues that stem from efforts to provide service to this unique population of families and children.

THE CHALLENGE FOR CHILDREN

An enduring and long range challenge for any child in substitute care is the issue of separation from, and loss of, the birth family. Helping children to cope with this experience is one of the most important tasks for health care and child welfare providers.

The most pressing clinical issue in regard to the hospitalized child is the concern about compromised development (Shore & Goldston, 1978). Often many of these children are developmentally delayed as a result of the original medical problems (Cohen, 1979; Sauve & Singhal, 1985; Yu, Orgill, Lim, Bajuk & Astbury, 1983). Specifically, hospitalization itself is viewed as a crisis which has a major negative impact on child development (Davis, Foster, Whitworth, & Skinner, 1982). The undesirable psychological and developmental effects of long term institutional care of infants was identified by Spitz (1945) long ago.

Body image is often an accompanying difficulty for this population. Actual body damage, physical anomalies and physical assaults from painful medical interventions may lead to negative body image, damaged self esteem and behavioral difficulty.

> J.V. consistently threw temper trantrums when first placed in foster care, creating a crisis and the need for nebulization treatments.

> K.E., a respirator-dependent child, still waiting for a family, disconnects his breathing tube, setting off alarms, as an attention seeking device. This behavior has had a deletrious impact on efforts to recruit foster families.

Peer relationships may suffer when children with special needs are surrounded by others with special needs in the hospital. This may be compounded within a foster home setting if the family, who has special skills, takes other medically complex or developmentally delayed children. It is further reinforced if they are placed in special education classrooms rather then mainstreamed with a broader range of children.

PRELIMINARY FINDINGS

The MFPP for transitioning medically complex children to the community is currently yielding data which demonstrate the developing effectiveness of this approach for some medically complex children; specifically for those children for whom a return to the birth families is not possible. The effectiveness of this program has been demonstrated by the successful transition of six children to community foster care. The cost effectiveness of this approach is also apparent.

Table 2 presents the cost of home care and hospital care for 6 MFPP children. Hospital costs ranged from $15,000 per month to $23,300 per month. This is based on Medicaid per diem rates which are fixed prospectively. These rates may not accurately reflect the actual cost of caring for these children i.e., costs are often higher than the fixed Medicaid reimbursement rates. Home care costs for these children ranged from $9,000 per month (D.F.) to $434 per month (the monthly board rate for specialized foster care). At the present time 2 children require only the monthly foster care board rate ($434), 3 require $100 per month, or less, for medical supplies in addition to the monthly foster care board rate and 1 child (D.F.) requires $9,000 per month for 16 hours per day of nursing care plus the monthly foster care board rate. Of note is the fact that several children (A.S. and J.H.) had high "up front" home care costs ($13,400

Table 12.1. Medical Foster Parent Program—Project Children.

Name	Age	Sex	Diagnosis	Duration in Hospital(s)	Duration in Project	Placement Status
R.W.	10 years	F	Spina Bifida	18 months	18 months	relative foster care
J.H.	2½ years	M	Vocal cord paralysis Tracheostomy	17 months	4 months	foster care
L.B.	3½ years	M	Bronchopulmonary dysplasia Tracheostomy	36+ months	14+ months	none found
O.M.	3½ years	M	Pierre Robin Syndrome Cleft palate	6 months	5 months	foster care
E.E.	3½ years	M	Bronchopulmonary dysplasia Tracheostomy	36+ months	12+ months	return home pending
D.F.	2+ years	F	Bronchopulmonary dysplasia Tracheostomy	25 months	12 months	foster care
J.V.	4 years	M	Bronchopulmonary dysplasia	8 months	7 months	foster care
L.R.	2½ years	M	Tracheostomy Subarachnoid hemorrhage Congenital syphilis Developmental delays Gastric tube	15+ months	8+ months	none found
K.E.	3½ years	M	Central hypoventilation syndrome Ventilator dependent Developmental delays	42+ months	18+ months	none found
T.W.	6½ years	M	Quadriplegic secondary to child abuse Ventilator dependent	19 months	6 months	pediatric nursing home foster placement pending
A.S.	3 years	M	Pierre Robin Syndrome Tracheostomy	28 months	10 months	foster care

Table 12.2. Cost of Hospital Care and Home Care.

Name	Duration of Hospitalization (in days)	Approximate Cost of Hospitalization[a]	Approximate Home Care Costs[b]
A.S.	850	$476,750 ($17,000/month)	$13,400/month for first 3 months. $434/month for foster care after the third month.
J.H.	525	$254,600 ($15,000/month)	$4,800/month for first month. $100/month + $434/month for foster care after the first month
D.F.	752	$476,000 ($18,000/month)	$9,000/month + $434/month for foster care
J.V.	229	$137,000 ($18,000/month)	$75/month + $434/month for foster care
O.M.	181	$122,000 ($20,300/month)	$434/month for foster care
R.W.	45	$22,000 ($15,000/month)	$75/month + $434/month for foster care

[a]Based on Medicaid per diem rates. Rates for 2 children (D.F. and J.V.) are blended i.e. Medicaid reimbursement rates changed during their hospitalization. Cost for 2 children (A.S. and D.F.) include 10 month stays at an acute care hospital.
[b]The State of Illinois pays $434/month to foster parents for children in specialized foster care. Payments are for food, clothing and shelter. Children receive a Medicaid card for medical expenses.

for the first 3 months of home care and $4,800 for the first month of home care, respectively). These relatively high initial home care costs were primarily for home nursing services. As the foster parents became more skilled at caring for the children themselves they requested, and in one instance demanded, the removal of home nursing services. The removal of home nursing services was done after a careful assessment of the parent(s) ability to adequately care for the child. These data reflect a marked cost savings for home care as opposed to hospital care for this, albeit small, population of children who have been successfully transitioned to the community.

This unique partnership between a pediatric hospital and a child welfare agency represents a specific systemic approach to the planning and service delivery problems faced by health care and child welfare professionals in a large, urban, setting. In developing this project a linear model for service between LRCH and CHASI was envisioned. It was anticipated that CHASI would be able to directly recruit all families for this population of children. The strong initial interest expressed by inexperienced families, and their subsequent failure to follow through with training and child placement, suggest that this is an overwhelming task requiring the skills of more experienced foster families. To recruit the requisite experienced foster families required the development of an expanded network of child welfare agencies. To effect the change from a linear model to a networking model, CHASI recruited experienced foster families from a wide array of cooperating child welfare agencies.

Overall, the value in this project has been not only the blending of the requisite health care and child welfare expertise, but also the identification of, and efforts to, reduce the systemic barriers which prohibit appropriate placement, funding and availability of community resources.

It is becoming increasingly clear that the challenge in transitioning this population rests with the ability of all systems to be committed, flexible, creative and aggressive in seeking to reduce barriers and arrive at solutions that will facilitate the transition to home care.

A review of the MFPP and the other models mentioned here, suggests that there are an array of responses, interventions and service delivery systems which can work in communities which are struggling to serve this population. There are a number of elements that appear to be essential to developing a community based foster care program for medically complex children. (1) Integration of health care and child welfare concepts is crucial. The process of transitioning these children to foster home placement is a remarkably complex undertaking requiring both health care and child welfare tasks. (2) Multidisciplinary planning and collaboration should include all essential systems to transition the child to the community (e.g. health care, social service, funding, school, home health care agencies, equipment vendors and others). (3) Professional networking should be undertaken as early in the transition process as possible. This will increase coordination of services to the population being served as well as expand opportunities for foster family recruitment. (4) It is essential to target recruitment efforts toward experienced foster families. For example, a local television feature story on the project generated twenty-eight new family referrals, none of which produced a viable family for project children. On the other hand, all four foster families who have received project children are experienced foster families. (5) Specialized training of foster parents is essential due to the complexities of the care required by these children. A standardized training program is important not only to impart the information necessary for the child's care but to reduce the apprehension associated with the responsibility. In addition to the standard curriculum, training specific to each child's individual needs is essential. (6) Family networking is a critical element in assisting families caring for this population. Networking facilitates support and mutual problem solving. The health care/child welfare partnership must encourage and participate in the development of this network. (7) Specialized training for all collaborating professionals is important due to the multidisciplinary nature of the tasks (e.g. social service personnel must learn medical terminology and home health care tasks to effectively assist foster parents). (8) Once the child is placed, ongoing services to the child, foster family, and birth family must be tailored to the individual needs of each (e.g. special education services, child and family therapy and case management).

The MFPP demonstrates that medically complex children who cannot be returned to their birth families can be transitioned successfully to community foster care. Ultimately, the challenge for the professional community in planning for this population rests with the successful development, acquisition and management of limited resources. This is one of the most persistent barriers which must be faced.

REFERENCES

Bieter, J. T., Kasbohm, R. K., Kaufmann, G. L., & Aufderheide, K. A. (1981). *The analysis of need for a pediatric transitional care resource in the Twin Cities area*. Minneapolis, MN: Hamilton Associates, Inc.

Cohen, M. M. (1979). Cleft palate, micrognathia and glossoptosis. In D. Bergsma (Ed.), *Birth defects compendium* (pp. 182). New York: Allen R. Liss, Inc.

Davis, A. B., Foster, P. H., & Whitworth, J. M. (1984). Medical foster care: A cost-effective solution to a community problem. *Child Welfare, 63*, 341–349.

Davis, A. B., Foster, P. H., Whitworth, J. M., & Skinner, R. G. (1982). Medical foster care: An alternative nursing practice. *Journal of Maternal Child Nursing, 7*, 245–248.

Department of Health and Human Services. (1986). *Medical foster care for seriously chronically medically ill children*. (Grant No. 90-CW-0790). Washington, D.C.: Office of Human Development Services, Administration for Children Youth and Families.

Dombro, R. H., & Haas, B. S. The chronically ill child and his family in the hospital. In M. Debuskey (Ed.), *The chronically ill child and his family* (pp. 163–180). Springfield, IL: Charles C. Thomas.

Education of the Handicapped Act of 1970, 20 U.S.C. 1400 (1975).

Gortmaker, S. (1985). Demography of chronic childhood diseases. In N. Hobbs & M. Perrin (Eds.), *Issues in the care of children with chronic illness* (pp. 135–154). San Francisco, CA: Josey-Bass.

Hobbs, N., Perrin, J. M., & Ireys, H. T. (1985). *Chronically ill children and their families.* San Francisco: Josey-Bass.

Kohrman, A. F. (1985, June). *Home health care for chronically ill children.* Paper presented to the U.S. Senate Committee on Labor and Human Relations. Washington, D.C.

Merkens, M. (1983). *Transitional care for chronically ill children.* Unpublished manuscript, La Rabida Children's Hospital, Chicago, Illinois.

Moos, R. H., & Tsu, B. D. (1977). The crisis of physical illness: An overview. In R. H. Moos (Ed.), *Coping with physical illness* (pp. 3–20). New York: Plenum Medical Book Company.

Newacheck, P. W., Budetti, P. T. & McManus, P. (1984). Trends in childhood disability, *American Journal of Public Health, 74,* 232–236.

Office of Technology Assessment (1987). *Technology-dependent children: Hospital v. home care—A technical memorandum* (Office of Technology Assessment, U.S. Congress, No. OTA-TM-H-38). Washington, D.C.: U.S. Government Printing Office.

Pierce, P. M., Freedman, S. A., & Reiss, J. G. (1987). Prescribed pediatric extended care (PPEC): A new link in the continuum. *Children's Health Care, 16,* 55–59.

Project Impact. (1984, April). Brochures and community education material. (Available from Project Impact, 25 West Street, Boston, MA).

Sauve, R. S., & Singhal, N. (1985). Long-term morbidity of infants with bronchopulmonary dysplasia. *Pediatrics, 76,* 725–733.

Shore, M., & Goldston, S. E. Mental health aspects of pediatric care. In P. Magrab (Ed.), *Psychological management of pediatric problems* (pp. 15–31), Baltimore, University Park Press.

Social Security Act of 1935, 602 U.S.C. 402 Title IV (1980).

Spitz, R. A. (1945). Hospitalism. In A. Freud, W. Hoffer, E. Glover, P. Greenacre, H. Hartman, E. B. Jackson, E. Kris, L. S. Kubie, B. Lewin, & M. C. Putnam (Eds.), *Psychoanalytic study of the child* (pp. 53–74). New York: International University Press.

Tekely, K., & Dittemore, I. (1978). Regressive behavior in a hospitalized pre-school child. *Maternal Child Nursing Journal, 7,* 185–190.

United Cerebral Palsy Association (1986, March). *The baby house.* (Available from the United Cerebral Palsy Association, Miami FL).

Vernon, D. T. A., Schulman, J. L., & Foley, J. M. (1966). Changes in children's behavior after hospitalization. *American Journal of Diseases of Children, 3,* 581–593.

Yu, V. H., Orgill, A. A., Lim, S. B., Bajuk, B. & Astbury, J. (1983). Growth and development of very low birth weight infants recovering from bronchopulmonary dysplasia. *Archives of Disease in Childhood, 58,* 791–794.

CHAPTER 13

COLLABORATION FOR FAMILIES

SARA MIRANDA
JANE QUINTON

INTRODUCTION

In November of 1984 the Massachusetts Departments of Mental Health, Public Health and Social Services entered into a unique partnership for the purpose of achieving permanent, nurturing family ties for children with developmental disabilities. This partnership involved these agencies in a three year demonstration project, the Collaboration for Families, sponsored by Project IMPACT, a private, non-profit special needs adoption agency.

This interagency project was supported through state funds and had as its goal addressing the findings of an earlier federally funded project, The Adoption Collaborative. The Adoption Collaborative, a jointly run program between the Developmental Evaluation Clinic at The Children's Hospital and Project IMPACT, found that the permanency planning needs of children with disabilities were significantly underserved in the state. Of the 1600 children with developmental disabilities in out-of-home care, 25–30% had no significant family involvement, a figure which remained consistent no matter which state agency held responsibility for the case. Additionally, scores of individual case studies indicated that those families who did have children with developmental disabilities were subject to a great deal of strain in keeping their children at home and had difficulty accessing or maintaining adequate support services (MARX, 1990). These children were therefore at risk of losing their existing family ties if parents felt they were unable to sustain the level of care required without supplemental supports from outside resources.

It was clear that with an explicit goal of permanency planning for children with disabilities—whether these children had no current family involvement or were in danger of losing what they had—the

Collaboration for Families needed to forge an interagency coalition. Only a joint commitment amongst agencies to keep or link children with families could provide the comprehensive planning and coordination necessary to create and implement family supports. The Adoption Collaborative recommended at its conclusion that the Departments of Mental Health, Public Health and Social Services work together on an interagency basis, using each other's expertise in order to insure permanent nurturing families for these children. The Department of Social Services would contribute knowledge of permanency planning, the Department of Mental Health would contribute its knowledge of normalization and developmental theory and the Department of Public Health its knowledge of physically handicapped children and health related community supports.

Before interagency cooperation could be effected specific systems barriers needed to be identified and recommendations for actions made. A series of task forces organized by the Collaboration for Families highlighted the following problem areas:

- *Lack of an articulated commitment to permanency planning for children with disabilities*, whether this lack emerged from an unfamiliarity with the concept (Department of Public Health) lack of sufficient knowledge of developmental disabilities (Department of Social Services).

- *Service gaps arising from the kind of service provision and delivery adopted by each agency.* The Department of Social Services used protective care issues to initiate service delivery, a mechanism which was not appropriate for many biological families who needed support services but had neither abused nor abandoned their children; the Department of Mental Health had no clear mandate to serve children; and the Department of Public Health had no provision for alternative family options to place a child out of home. The practical consequence of these delineations was that it was nearly impossible to coordinate services across agencies. Thus, if a child were in an institution he or she received little or no permanency planning, or if a child were still in his or her family the family received few support services to ease the challenges to routine functioning.

- *Disproportionate allotment of funds to out-of-home care rather than family support.* Funding continued to be geared toward institutional care rather than to supporting families, giving the unspoken message that it is preferable to place children with disabilities out of home.

The least support went to families who kept their children at home and there was little recognition of the need for ongoing support services for those families.

• *Lack of creative models for providing family based options to children*, such as co-parenting, visiting resources, routine respite care, specialized foster care and open adoption. Although creative alternatives had been developed by some individual line workers on a case by case basis there were no programs set up to specifically respond to the needs of children and families in these cases. Ideally, a range of options could be offered as alternatives; however, pursuing such options would require an integrated and flexible approach to providing services and coordinating resources amongst all of the agencies involved.

Once these barriers were identified the Collaboration was able to outline and implement a four tiered strategy for meeting the permanency planning needs of developmentally disabled children. This strategy included establishing a network of work groups which involved staff from all three state agencies, a program of training and development for workers at these agencies, a jointly endorsed position paper outlining each agencies permanency planning philosophy (Quinton & Martin, 1987) and a direct service component. The direct service component was staffed by two full-time social workers, one of whom recruited visiting resources, weekend families and/or legal guardians for young adults in institutions and the other who took on casework and family support responsibilities for 8–10 developmentally disabled children. The efforts of the former have been described in a separate publication, *Somebody Special* (Schroen, 1987). The work of the latter is described below.

CASEWORK SERVICES TO FAMILIES

One objective of this direct service component of the Collaboration was to identify the skills needed to work with the families of children with multiple disabilities. A second objective was to develop more flexible family options for these children. The worker who was selected brought with her an extensive background in developmental disabilities gained through hospital experience, as well as a knowledge of working with families around medically related issues.

During the first three years of the program, 19 children received direct services through this contract. This included five young children in hospital settings, five children who had always been cared for at home, four in long term foster homes and five children and adolescents in residential settings. The majority of cases involved multiple handicaps or severe medical problems, requiring significant in-home health care. Half of the cases involved either suctioning, g-tube feedings, tracheostomy care, catheterization, oxygen administration, and/ or heart monitors.

The Collaboration served parents who sought voluntary services, as well as parents who were referred because of protective issues. All cases involved a child whose family ties were at risk and whose parents needed help in identifying and following through on a plan for permanency.

Although each situation was unique, all of the families had been impacted by the birth of a handicapped child. In spite of disparate cultural backgrounds and social situations, these families shared a common struggle in attempting to adjust to the birth and long term care needs of their children. Elements of this struggle included grieving for the loss of the hoped for "perfect" child and accepting the reality of the disability, explaining the situation to relatives, friends and professionals, obtaining specialized medical and educational services, managing the daily care of a severely handicapped child, and planning for the future.

Assessment

All cases which were accepted by the Collaboration began with an assessment by the caseworker. The assessment included observation of the child in as many settings as possible. Information was gathered from parents, respite and substitute care providers, and medical and educational personnel.

Our experience underscored the importance of using a worker who had a good knowledge base in developmental disabilities and who felt comfortable interacting with a severely handicapped child. The worker needed to be able to assess the child's strengths as well as the nature and extent of the disability. The worker also gathered information on the child's functioning on several levels, including cognitive, perceptual, motor and emotional.

It was also important to determine the meaning a child held for his or her family. What was the level of interaction between the child and various family members? Who had the primary caretaking role?

Was the child successful in communicating his or her needs? How had the family's lifestyle changed since the birth of the child? What emotional supports were available to the family? How did parents view their future with this child? Answers to these questions helped shape the direction of a permanent plan.

As part of a psychosocial evaluation, the assessment addressed the daily concrete demands placed on a family by a disabled child. How many hours of general and specialized care were needed? Were the parents able to obtain sufficient outside help through respite workers, home health aides, or nurses? What were the needs for specialized equipment and medical supplies? Were supplies, equipment and respite adequately funded by insurance, SSI or Medicaid? Was the family's income being depleted? Was the home fully accessible for a handicapped child? Answers to these questions helped the worker to clarify the family's situation and to understand how a child who was clearly loved by parents could still be a source of stress and ambivalence.

Casework Practice

Casework with families who had multiply handicapped children required clinical skills as well as a knowledge base pertaining to disability. Clinical skills were critical in helping parents sort out the elements of their dilemma and in enabling them to make informed choices necessary for a permanent plan.

These skills were also critical in helping develop a relationship between the worker and parents, and the importance of establishing a viable relationship with parents cannot be overemphasized. Cases referred to the Collaboration most often involved distressed families in crisis. A positive relationship with the worker aided parents in relaxing, in disclosing information, and in beginning to trust that a solution was possible.

Relationship building began during the assessment phase. An initial contact with parents was used to explain the worker's role, to outline responsibilities, and to briefly review options. The rationale for permanency planning was explained at this time. Although parents were usually not able to fully integrate or discuss the options at the outset of the case, it was imperative to be open and frank with the family from the very beginning. As the case progressed and parents were able to trust the worker, options were continually reviewed.

Respect for the families and children and a non-judgmental attitude were essential in helping the worker maintain an empathic, but neutral stance. Families who felt they could not bring a handicapped infant home were accorded the same respect as families who had been struggling for years to maintain a child at home. In cases where families needed to surrender the child, the decision was always seen as valid. The worker's role was to help achieve a permanent plan for the child, not to make moral judgments. Each family presented different strengths and different tolerances for stress. The goal, however, was always to provide the child with a strong family tie and the worker sometimes helped families decide whether it was possible to keep that child with them. For those families where out of home placement was not the issue the worker needed to remember that her appraisal of a particular child's appeal was not the issue. Families' perceptions of their children's attractiveness and responsiveness remained the important factor.

Most families required validation, both for their efforts on the child's behalf and in reinforcing the importance and value of their particular child. Relationships with parents were enhanced by the worker's interaction with the child, observation of the child, and understanding that the child's progress was often reflected in small increments.

Frequent contact and worker accessibility were factors in establishing a good relationship. The worker often accompanied parents to a medical appointment, case conference or school evaluation and visited the home regularly. Distressed parents often benefited from telephone contact with the worker.

Contact with the worker allowed families to experience some emotional relief through the telling and retelling of their child's "story." Ventilation of feelings was a necessary step, and the worker needed to feel comfortable with a parent's strong emotions. Universalization was also important at this time. Parents clearly benefited from the knowledge that other families had undergone similar experiences. Guilt was alleviated by letting parents know that anger and feelings of helplessness were common reactions.

Ambivalence in decision making played a part in every case. At times, families seemed to go backward, changing their focus and reversing decisions. The worker needed to remain empathic while helping parents move forward.

All parents were encouraged to consider the pros and cons of various placement options for their child. The worker talked with parents about the importance of parental involvement for children and the impact which long term residential care or foster care can have on children. Families learned about the support services available to them. Some chose to talk with a parent of a child with a similar disability. They also learned about a range of available options. When appropriate, they were given information about the adoption process, including the information that children find adoptive homes more readily when they are young. Within the context of a relationship with a case-worker whom they trusted, most families were able to use this information and make decisions which they considered best for their children.

Concrete service plans with specific tasks and time lines for completion were essential. The actual length of a case varied, but most were completed in a six to fourteen month period. Although it was necessary to help parents make decisions in a timely manner, rushing parents through the process was not seen as productive.

Case Management

Case management skills were important in helping families make permanent plans. The most common need was for help with the child in the family home, whether through respite workers, home health aides, or nurses. Out-of-home respite was also frequently requested. Many families required aid in obtaining medical supplies, specialized equipment, ramps and lifts to make the home accessible. Funding for equipment and services was often problematic for families. Advocacy and help in negotiating systems such as Medicaid and Supplemental Social Security Insurance became standard practice.

At times it was necessary to refer parents for individual or family therapy. Referrals reflected the worker's assessment that ongoing problems in the family could not be adequately addressed within this service model alone. Referrals were made to obtain behavior management for siblings, psychotherapy for a parent, and consultation from a child psychiatrist to help parents inform their children of a decision to surrender a sibling.

Protective Cases

A number of the cases referred to the Collaboration involved issues of emotional and physical neglect. In these cases the worker assessed whether parents could provide a minimum sufficient level of care to ensure a child's health and well being. Often the worker needed to determine whether it was the demands of the child's handicap or a lack of parenting ability that led to the neglect situation. In some cases it was useful to refer the child for a comprehensive evaluation. The evaluation helped to determine whether a child's medical problems and low functioning level were organically based or a result of neglect.

Protective cases usually had substantial involvement by a Department of Social Services worker. A "team" approach was used, with the Collaboration worker and the Department of Social Services worker jointly meeting with parents. This helped decrease "splitting" by parents and ensured that both workers gave the same message to a family. The workers also shared responsibility for case documentation and for writing service plans and case reviews.

It was essential that service plans written for protective cases were detailed and concrete. Tasks for parents were always linked to a specific time frame. Tasks included specific training in a child's disability, attendance at parenting classes, and participation in school meetings and medical appointments.

Specialized foster care was used in cases where parents were not able to meet a child's needs. In these cases, regular visitation was part of the plan. Specialized foster care provided the child with a safe, nurturing environment, while parents worked on tasks to enable them to resume caretaking.

A six month period was usually sufficient to determine the direction of a protective case. If termination of parental rights appeared to be the only alternative, the Department of Social Services' worker scheduled legal and clinical conferences and began the termination process.

Specialized Foster Care

Specialized foster care was used in both protective and voluntary cases. Foster care was always seen as temporary, and as a means of helping parents to make a decision regarding a permanent plan.

In voluntary cases, specialized foster care was offered when parents appeared overwhelmed by the demands of their disabled child and needed a lengthy respite or a time to focus on decision-making. Specialized foster care was also useful for those parents with a very medically involved, young child who had always resided in an acute care setting. Parents who had never seen their child cared for outside of a hospital unit needed to see "proof" that the child's care could be managed in a home. Foster parents were able to teach these families specifics about the child's daily care and to model appropriate ways of handling the child.

Birth parents had mixed reactions to the suggestion that a period of specialized foster care be used. Some parents were enthusiastic about foster care and wanted this as a permanent arrangement. Parents were always informed of the temporary nature of substitute care—usually six months to one year. The worker would review permanency planning philosophy at this time, explaining that foster care did not constitute a permanent, legal commitment to the child. Parents were reminded that disruptions in long-term foster care were common, particularly when a multi-handicapped child reached adolescence and become more difficult to manage physically. Birth parents were also told that as the foster parents themselves grew older, decisions to move or to retire were possible. The worker's goal was to help parents realize that "permanent" foster care was not in the child's best interest and that only return home, guardianship or adoption could provide permanency.

Some birth parents had very strong objections to foster care, preferring the child to be placed in a residential setting. Overcoming a prejudicial reaction to foster care involved substantial education. The worker explained that specialized foster care involved people who were highly skilled and very committed to providing quality care for handicapped children. At times parents required reassurance that their child would not forget them or transfer affection to the new caretakers.

The Collaboration worker was responsible for locating and supervising the specialized foster placement. The foster parents were seen as skilled professionals who could offer a special service to the child. Many had adopted and/or fostered several children with developmental disabilities and medical involvement. Most specialized foster parents had some formal training in managing the care of multi-handicapped children.

It was important to provide support and case management services for foster parents. As the care for multi-handicapped children was complex and time consuming, it was essential that specialized foster parents receive adequate payment. Case management also involved helping foster parents access services for the child.

Although most foster parents worked quite well with birth parents, there were situations when foster parents felt uncomfortable or defensive in response to birth parents. The worker needed to promote communication between foster and birth parents and to defuse any hostile feeling. At times, the worker also needed to help foster parents understand that birth parents who placed or surrendered children, had valid reasons for doing so.

Foster parents were expected to allow visitation by birth parents. Usually, the visitation took place in the foster home. If birth parents were problematic in any way, the worker supervised each visit.

Permanency Options

The goal of the Collaboration for Families program was to secure a permanent family tie for each child who was referred. This goal allowed the caseworker to support the biological parents' choice of several options. Options included maintaining a child at home or returning a child home, surrender for closed adoption or for open adoption, and legal guardianship. In certain situations, the use of visiting resources was also an appropriate option. The decision to maintain a child at home or to bring a child home from a residential facility or hospital was made by several families.

Families who felt that no amount of services would be sufficient to keep a child at home, were usually able to choose the option of surrender for adoption. In most cases, the adoption was closed, with no contact between birth parents and child following the surrender. Closed (confidential, no contact between parties) adoption provided the largest pool of potential adoptive parents for a child, as most potential families were uncomfortable with the idea of continued contact with birth parents. For some birth families, closed adoption also provided a feeling of closure. Some birth families also left a letter in the case record, requesting that the adoptive family send a yearly progress note to the agency.

Families who maintained a relationship and ongoing contact with an older child in substitute care, were able to surrender the child for an open adoption. Open adoption (some contact between parties) provided a means of establishing permanency for the child, with an opportunity to retain the prior parental relationship. Open adoption did restrict the number of potential adoptive families. A contract which detailed visiting arrangements was completed prior to the surrender. Visits by birth families were limited to 3 to 4 times a year. This arrangement required careful social work planning and intervention and was used only in circumstances where the child could clearly benefit.

Legal guardianship was another option for parents who had maintained an ongoing relationship with their child, but could not manage the child at home. The arrangement provides the child with greater permanency than foster care, while allowing contact with the biological family. A written visiting plan and careful delineation of rights and responsibilities for both families must be built into the arrangement.

Although the vast majority of permanent plans led to placement in a family setting, a few children required ongoing residential placement. One child benefited from care in a pediatric nursing home as the family's situation prevented them from caring for the child on a full time basis. In this case the family tie was supported by helping the family formulate a written visiting plan. Three adolescents living in residential facilities were referred to the Collaboration for a visiting resource. They needed volunteer families who could visit, provide advocacy and offer their homes on vacations and weekends. The pool of potential visiting families was limited, and innovative recruitment techniques were needed to locate families.

CONCLUSION

The goal of the Collaboration for Families in providing direct services was to demonstrate the range of permanent plans available to children with developmental disabilities and the casework services necessary to achieve these plans. Of the nineteen children referred by the Department of Social Services, ten were voluntarily surrendered for adoption and are now with permanent families. Three biological families chose to maintain their severely medically involved children at home. Two other families chose residential placement with a commitment to visit their children regularly. The Department of Social Services has initiated procedures to terminate parental rights for two children who have been placed in legal risk adoptive families. One family has chosen a co-parenting arrangement with weekly overnight visits. Visiting families were recruited for three adolescents in residential care.

Permanency planning needs to be adapted for this population to allow for more flexibility of family options. Major ingredients in achieving successful outcomes are the worker's skills and attitude, a caseload small enough to allow for intensive family work and sufficient community supports to enable these children to be cared for in family settings.

REFERENCES

Marx, J. (1990). Better me than somebody else: Families reflect on their adoption of developmentally disabled children. In L. Glidden (Ed.), *Formed Families: Adoption of Children with Handicaps* (pp 166–173). New York: Haworth Press.

Quinton, J., & Martin, S. (1987). *Permanency planning for children with developmental disabilities*. (Available from [Project Impact, 25 West Street, Boston, MA, 02111]).

Schroen, S. (1987). *Somebody special: The family resource program at the Hogan Regional Center*. (Available from [Project Impact, 25 West Street, Boston, MA, 02111]).

CHAPTER 14

SPECIALIZED FOSTER CARE FOR CHILDREN WITH HIV

PHYLLIS GURDIN
GARY R. ANDERSON

INTRODUCTION

In the mid-1980s New York City was facing a new and frightening medical and child welfare crisis. As a byproduct of the proliferation of crack, a readily attainable affordable derivative of cocaine, high numbers of young women were giving birth to infants addicted to cocaine. In addition to the medical and behavioral complications of this addiction, infants were being left in the hospital by parents who were too ill or disorganized to care for the newborn, or the infants were prevented from returning to their parents by authorities concerned about child neglect and maltreatment. The term "boarder baby" became applied to this population, over 300 infants each month, remaining in the hospital past the time of medical necessity and with no place to go. The number of beds in the foster care system had been shrinking in size and consequently was unprepared for a major influx of infants needing placement.

A subset of this special needs population posed a particular challenge—infants who tested positive for the Human Immunodeficiency Virus (HIV) associated with Acquired Immunodeficiency Syndrome (AIDS) [Anderson, 1984]. An increase in infants with HIV was linked to the use of drugs, particularly crack, due to the use of unclean needles shared for intravenous injections of drugs and raising money to support a demanding drug habit by having multiple sex partners. These high risk behaviors among women of child bearing age, in addition to women having sex with drug abusing, potentially infected men, resulted in high numbers of young children with HIV infection and AIDS. New York City has consistently accounted for a significant number of reported pediatric AIDS cases in the United States—706 of the 2,686 cumulative cases reported to the Centers for Disease Control [CDC, 1990].

Dr. John Hutchings, Assistant Director of the Division of Maternal and Child Health, Department of Health and Human Services, expressed common concerns about boarder babies:

> The babies who are left in hospitals should be placed in homes for two good reasons. One, no matter how concerned and loving the hospital staff is, a home environment is still recognized as the best place for a child. There is a more stable environment in the home, and not such a crowd of people hovering over the baby. Also socialization with other children, if it is possible or appropriate, is very important for the child. Two, the cost of hospital care to the state and public is enormous." [Gentry, 1985]

For children with HIV infection, there often were not so many people "hovering over the baby" as fear of AIDS resulted in isolation or approaching the young children garbed in surgical gowns, mask, and gloves.

Beginning a Foster Care Program

Discharging HIV-infected infants into a typical foster home was not working. Foster parents refused to accept these children, and oftentimes when the HIV was discovered after a placement was made the child would be returned to the hospital by the distressed foster parents. The need for a specialized program became clear due to this stigma, increasing numbers of children, and the need for specialized services.

At the request of city and state officials, Leake and Watts Children's Home, a respected 159-year-old New York City multi-service child caring agency working with over 1,500 city children in several types of congregate care and foster families, began a foster care program for HIV children. With strong board and administrative support, and initial funding from the AIDS Institute of the New York State Health Department, the program began to recruit, train and work with foster parents.

Recruitment and Homefinding

Finding a sufficient number of foster parents to care for children with HIV was an initial and ongoing challenge. Recruitment efforts have included speaking to numerous community and professional groups, advertisements and public service announcements, and appeals to special populations (such as persons with a medical background who may be less intimidated by the medical needs of children). The most effective method of recruitment has been networking through existing foster parents. The first homes for this program were located by asking foster parents in the Leake and Watts boarding home program to suggest friends and relatives who might be good candidates for specialized foster care. After a core of foster parents was recruited to the program, they have become key resources in sharing their experiences with prospective parents and in identifying others who might be interested in foster parenting [Gurdin & Anderson, 1987].

After an initial recruitment phase, an intake and homefinding process begins. This stage examines the quality of the home and the parent's understanding of the potential work with a HIV + child. The need for foster parents has not resulted in a "watering down" of the expectations for caring for a child. A number of criteria for accepting an applicant have been identified.

- There should be no other foster children in the home and no biological children under the age of six, due to the risk of infecting the seropositive child.

- All members of the family must be informed and accept medical explanations for HIV transmission and be willing to care for the child.

- Parents must recognize that a child will often be sick and they will have to accompany the child on numerous medical appointments, must accept the possibility of the child having developmental delays and/or emotional problems, and in some cases, the child may die.

- A responsible member of the family must be available in the home or a proven support system of friends or relatives to supervise the child must be in place.

- Family members must prioritize the care of the foster child and be willing to work as team members with agency staff members.

- Although not crucial, a basic knowledge of medical principles and treatment by one family member is helpful due to required compliance with medical care instructions and the need for prompt attention to conditions that may precede or indicate an emergency [Gurdin 1989].

The foster parents for this program, now numbering over 60 homes, have a number of key qualities in common: (1) prior knowledge of HIV and AIDS so that this program was not the first time they had been confronted with the issue of AIDS, (2) confidence that they were not at risk of acquiring AIDS by caring for HIV+ children, and (3) often, past personal or family experience with chronic illness. Prospective foster parents expressed a desire to take care of an HIV-infected child, rather than a child with other needs.

The Placement Process

A child enters the foster care program from one of two routes—either directly from a hospital referred by a city child welfare worker based in the hospital or from transitional residences for HIV+ infants in the city that serve as a bridge between hospitalization and foster home location. Transitional residences are group homes for young children that have beds for HIV-infected children who do not require hospitalization but for whom an appropriate foster home has not yet been located. These residences reduce the time children stay in hospital settings, and in a more home-like environment take care of children, assess their needs, and begin to reach out to biological families.

Through direct placement or a transitional residence, the program's first action is to assess the medical, developmental, and psychosocial needs of the child. This assessment is conducted by program nurses and social workers and is based on observation, consultations with medical and social service personnel presently involved with the child, and by reading charts and case notes.

Children present with a variety of medical conditions related to HIV infection: (1) small size for their age; (2) failure to thrive; (3) generalized swelling of lymph glands; (4) different types of pneumonia; (5) chronic diarrhea; (6) recurrent viral and bacterial infections; (7) thrush; (8) opportunistic infections, such as pneumocystis carinii pneumonia; (9) other evidence of immune system suppression [Rendon, Gurdin, Bassi, & Weston, 1989]. In addition to these medical conditions the temperament, behavior, and developmental appropriateness of the child is assessed by the agency psychologist using anthropometric measurements and a variety of scales (for example, Merrill-Palmer Scale, Bailey Psychomotor Developmental Index, Bailey Mental Developmental Index, Wechsler Intelligence Scale for Children). These factors are important as it can be discouraging for foster parents to have children who are either too severely ill or developmentally and emotionally retarded so that no amount of loving care and expert assistance will have positive results for the infant. This assessment and prognosis may be difficult to make as young infants have been in institutional environments for most of their lives and are often recovering from neonatal addictions, so the potential impact of a home environment with consistent nurturance from parent may be difficult to project.

If the child is considered appropriate for the program, the potential foster parent is informed of the child's condition and the foster parent may meet the child in the institution before a placement is finalized. On the day the child is moved to the foster home, the child is transported by the program nurse to the home allowing the foster parent another opportunity to be ready for the child's entrance. When a child is accepted into the program the staff members also begin efforts to locate the child's parents and relatives.

PROGRAM DESCRIPTION

The program began with ten children and eight foster parents, the program has expanded to 64 foster parents caring for 90 children. This expansion in children served has been paralled by a growing staff team, an increasing range of services, and involvement with children and their foster families from across the city.

Staff Members

The first staff member was the program director, who came to the agency with over twenty years of experience in child welfare. Her early mandate was to begin this specialized program and this included performing all essential roles, such as recruiting foster parents, locating and placing children, working with the foster parents, reaching out to biological parents, building and supervising a staff team, fund raising, and public relations. The second staff person, a foster parent recruiter, joined the director in initial tasks of speaking to audiences, networking with existing AIDS agencies (such as Gay Mens' Health Crisis) primarily addressing the adult population, recruitment and training of foster parents, and supervising placements. The ongoing task of work with foster parents and children has been done by staff nurse and social worker teams who regularly visit with foster families, reach out to biological families, and respond to crises. The hiring of a nurse and social worker filled out the initial staff team; the program's expansion has been accompanied by adding nurses and social workers to the program, as well as administrative and supervisory personnel.

A crucial linkage that has provided necessary resources for the program has been a partnership with major medical institutions and its pediatric and AIDS-related clinics and specialists (for example, Albert Einstein Medical Center, Bronx Lebanon, and New York Hospital). The children located in the region have been followed by the hospital teams, providing necessary medical treatment and supplementing the counseling, education and supervision provided by the program staff team. The program has also benefited from a high level of cooperation and assistance from the city's Child Welfare Administration and the New York State Department of Social Services, who have provided resources needed by the program.

Program Services

The recruitment and sustainment of foster parents is enabled by an array of program services provided by program staff or secured from collateral sources. Initial services to foster families include education with regard to HIV, infection control, confidentiality issues, and the multiple needs of HIV children in general, and the needs of their child in particular. This education is provided primarily through the one-to-one relationship of nurse or social worker to foster parent. In addition to this relationship, there are support group meetings and more formal training on issues of common concern to the foster parents. Social workers typically have a caseload of 12 children; registered nurses work with as many as 15 children. Staff members are on-call twenty-four hours a day, every day. Although this after-hours availability is not frequently used, there have been times when foster parents have sought advice or support, or have reported a sudden change in the child's medical condition. When a foster parent has to take a child to the hospital or for a medical appointment they are usually accompanied by a staff nurse.

One of the primary needs of foster parents is acquiring the concrete items that they might need to care for the child. These needs include diapers, infant furniture, clothes, and in some cases such major items as washing machines—the agency will supply or assist in acquiring whatever is needed to appropriately care for the child. The funds for these concrete items come from a combination of public agency support and private donations.

Ongoing medical care is typically provided by a pediatric AIDS specialized clinic associated with a New York City Medical Center within close proximity to the foster home. Support, encouragement and guidance for foster families is provided by program social workers, nurses, the director, the foster parents themselves, medical social workers and other community resources. These organizationally-linked relationships are in addition to the family and informal supports that foster families have found to be helpful and sympathetic to their caring for a special child who may be stigmatized by some in the community. In some cases, foster families have relied on agency relationships as concerns about confidentiality and discrimination have limited the effectiveness of informal support networks.

An important aspect of this program that is receiving increased attention is respite care. Foster parents need some relief to take care of personal business, rest and relax, or spend special time with their biological children. Respite care for this program has usually involved asking the foster family to identify a key person to assist the family, with the agency paying for this babysitting arrangement. Some foster parents have used more formal channels for finding assistance, including home health aides supplied by local agencies. Committing resources to provide respite care is crucial as having recruited families it is essential that they be supported and encouraged to provide high quality care. This is only possible if they have some moments of relief. Anxiety of anticipation of illness and fear of the future is an ongoing challenge. Despite the stress from the demands of this type of child care, no foster parents have withdrawn from this specialized program to date.

There are a number of special services that can assist and enrich the foster parenting. Some children and their foster parents have participated in special camp programs designed for children with HIV and their caregivers, such as Camp Sunburst in California. Initial explorations for a local camp program have been initiated by some personnel from a Bronx medical center. A number of children are enrolled in the day care center at the Bronx Municipal hospital, that provides transportation, education, and support for children and families. Many are involved in formal foster parent support groups. With city support, there are annual events to express official gratitude for the foster parents. Although the foster parents receive an enriched

board rate for caring for this specialized group of special needs children ($1231 a month per child), these funds cannot begin to com-
pensate families for the love, commitment, time and energy that they
devote to the children.

City Involvement

There are over 400 HIV+ children in foster care agencies in New
York City, in addition to the 90 at Leake and Watts. With the financial
support provided by a grant from the Office of Human Development
Services, Department of Health and Human Services, the Leake and
Watts program has become a resource to other city child welfare
agencies who do not have specialized programs for children with HIV
infection. This outreach and support is provided in conjunction with
the New York State Department of Social Services.

Some examples of services provided by this federally-funded project include:

- A hotline number for foster parents and child welfare workers who
  need information, referrals, or guidance related to HIV and children.

- A consultation service in which staff members meet with other
  personnel from other agencies to discuss problems in service delivery or developing resources for foster families and children.

- An educational outreach initiative for professional and community
  groups to provide HIV education and present the needs of children,
  their families, and other caregivers.

- The initiation of regional support groups for foster parents from a
  number of agencies who may be feeling that they are alone or
  isolated while caring for an HIV+ child.

- The publication of a newsletter providing up-to-date medical information, resource information, and news of value to foster parents
  and child welfare workers alike.

- The publication of issue specific guidelines—addressing such issues
  as homefinding and recruitment, and respite care.

- The sharing of information and experiences with a wide audience
  of professionals and community persons through participation in
  regional and national conferences, workshops, and forums.

CURRENT ISSUES

A number of issues have posed a particular challenge to this program, for example:

(1) the *uncertainty of diagnosis* when many infants are tested and identified as HIV+ in their first year yet some will seroconvert at approximately age 15–18 months and then test negative for HIV antibodies. The initial positive test was due to the presence of the mother's antibodies—indicating that the mother was HIV-infected. But not all children born to an HIV+ mother will retain and develop their own HIV infection. Some of these seroconverted children, however, are more ill and troubled than some of the children who remain HIV+.

(2) the *complication in care* posed by the effects of neonatal drug addiction as many of these children acquired HIV from mothers who were drug users during their pregnancies [Blakeslee, 1989]. In this respect, there are common issues with HIV+ children and the larger number of boarder baby children with special needs due to drug exposure.

(3) the *desire of many foster families to adopt* their foster children which requires a certain amount of time and legal preparation that can be frustrating to eager parents concerned about the future of their foster children.

(4) the need to *cope with the death of children* in care. Although there have been only nine deaths, and these children had been brought into care in relatively sick condition and died soon after placement, there is a special grief that comes from the death of a young child. Each death also confronts the ongoing denial of death which may often be necessary to maintain a hopeful involvement with one's HIV infected child. Yet original predictions of numerous dying children have not yet proven true as children are living longer than ever expected and this has posed a challenge for the program as children grow older and approach school age.

CONCLUSION

The demands and anxieties of providing care for children with HIV are more than offset by the numerous examples of children who have thrived in loving homes. Although expectations must be realistic and handicapping conditions accepted, foster parents have been able to see and have contributed to the health and growth of many children. These children may have faced shorter and less quality of a life without the commitment of a family.

This program has demonstrated that it is possible to find parents to care for HIV-infected children, provide consistent medical care and loving attention, and find their own lives enriched as they nurture children who may have begun life with difficult circumstances to overcome. As increasing numbers of HIV + children are identified, and as other children, with or without the virus become orphaned as parents die from AIDS, the need to provide compassionate care for children will need to be replicated, refined, and distributed across this country.

REFERENCES

Anderson, G. R. (1984). Children and AIDS: Implications for Child Welfare. *Child Welfare, 63*, 62–73.

Blakeslee, S. (1989, September 17). Crack's Toll Among Babies: A Joyless View, Even of Toys. *New York Times*, p. 1.

Centers for Disease Control (1990). AIDS Cases and Annual Incidence Rates, Table 2. *HIV/AIDS Surveillance*. November. 7.

Gentry, L. (1985). AIDS Babies-Walls Around Children? *Colorado's Children, 4*, 4.

Gurdin, P. (1989). *Homefinding Guidelines for HIV-Seropositive Children*. (Available from Leake and Watts Children's Home, 487 South Broadway, Suite 201, Yonkers, New York 10705).

Gurdin, P. & Anderson, G. R. (1987). Quality Care for Ill Children: AIDS-Specialized Foster Family Homes. *Child Welfare, 66*, 291–302.

Rendon, M., Gurdin, P., Bassi, J., & Weston, M. (1989). Foster Care for Children with AIDS: A Psychosocial Perspective. *Child Psychiatry and Human Development, 19*, 256–269.

Section VII

Other Critical Issues: Legal, Ethical and Funding

CHAPTER 15

LEGAL ADVOCACY FOR MEDICALLY COMPLEX CHILDREN IN FOSTER CARE

MARK C. WEBER*

INTRODUCTION

This chapter addresses legal issues involved in obtaining services for foster families with medically complex children. Health and social work professionals frequently act as advocates for foster families in the families' efforts to get income support and social services, medical care, and education from public and private providers. Knowledge of legal entitlements can be the key to obtaining these services.

Although the body of this chapter deals with legal rights and procedures, two points must be made at the outset about the process of legal advocacy itself. The first is that, just as in the health care field, sometimes the best help a professional can provide is assistance for the client in obtaining the help of someone else. Lists of providers of free or low cost legal assistance are available from local bar associations; in the field of special education they are also available from the state educational agency. Persons not licensed to practice law should not dispense legal advice or attempt to represent others before courts or other entities that restrict representatives to those who have a law license.

The second point is that anyone acting as an advocate must avoid conflicts of interest among the persons being helped. This problem may be acute in a foster family setting, for the child's interests may be at odds with those of the foster parent or those of the natural parent. For example, a foster parent may want to keep an older foster

*The author would like to thank Andre LaBerge of the DePaul University College of Law for his able research assistance.

child in the house to help in the care of younger children, but the older child may have an interest in rapid transition to independence or a group home setting. There may even be conflicts between the interests of the child or the parent as they express them and the interests as the health or social work professional perceives them. The foster child may desperately want to live independently, but the professional may consider the goal unrealistic and prefer that the child have a longer period in foster care with eventual transition to a group home.

Regarding the issue of conflicts between clients, recommended attorney conduct guidelines of the American Bar Association (1983, Rule 1.7) prohibit representation of a client if the representation is directly adverse to that of another client or if the representation of one client is materially limited by that of the other. Conflicting representation is permissible only under the unlikely circumstance that the representation will not adversely affect either client and the clients consent after full consultation.

The implication is that the advocate must decide whom to represent: foster parent, natural parent, or child. Natural parents and foster parents are entitled to make some decisions on the child's behalf, but the advocate who acts on the basis of those decisions represents parent, not child. A guardian appointed by a court has authority to make some types of decisions on the ward's behalf, but typically the foster parent is not a guardian. The child's guardian is likely to be a child welfare agency, and frequently the agency has budgetary and bureaucratic interests that are inimical to those of the child.

There is no obvious solution to the problems involved in representing persons whose expressed needs conflict with their apparent needs. The American Bar Association guidelines (1983, Rule 1.14) state that when immaturity, mental disability, or other conditions impair a client's ability to make adequately considered decisions in connection with the representation, the attorney must, as far as reasonably possible, maintain a normal client-lawyer relationship. In a normal client-lawyer relationship, the client makes the decisions about important matters. Nevertheless, the guidelines recognize that deferring to the client may not be possible under some circumstances.

The remainder of this chapter covers three areas in which knowledge of legal rights and procedures is likely to assist persons advocating for a medically complex child or for the child's foster parent: income maintenance and social services, medical care, and special education. Hardin (1983) and Horowitz, Harden and Bulkley (1989) provide a detailed discussion of legal issues that may affect all foster children, such as emergency custody hearings, neglect and abuse proceedings, termination of parental rights, long-term planning, parental visitation, return of children to natural parents, adoption, and group litigation under the adoption assistance law.

INCOME MAINTENANCE AND SOCIAL SERVICES ISSUES

Foster parents receive payments for the children under their care. Medically complex children ordinarily qualify for specialized foster care payments, which are higher than regular foster care amounts. Monthly medical subsidy payments from the state agency give additional financial support. Typically, private social services agencies provide a package of funding and social services for the children they serve. The rates established by the state agency may permit private agencies to pay amounts that exceed those the state agency pays on direct contract with foster parents. State statutes or regulations lay out the methods by which the state agency sets payment levels (e.g., Illinois Administrative Code, 1988); wide variations in payment levels exist among states. Federal law requires that states must review the payment levels at reasonable intervals to ensure their continued appropriateness (Code of Federal Regulations, Title 45, § 1356.21(g)(1), 1989). Hearings must be provided to a foster parent or child whose claim for payments or other benefits is denied or not acted upon promptly (Title 45, § 1355.30(k), 1989).

With respect to social services, the Adoption Assistance and Child Welfare Act of 1980, sometimes referred to as Public Law 96-272, makes foster children generally eligible for social services under Title XX of the Social Security Act (1935) and requires that states furnish foster children with particularized services to reunify them with their natural families in accordance with a case plan for each child. The case plan is a written document with a description of the child's placement, a discussion of its appropriateness, a plan for ensuring that the child receives proper care, and a plan for services to the natural parents, child, and foster parents to improve the conditions in the natural parents' home and otherwise facilitate return of the child to that home or placement in a permanent setting.

The plan must be designed to achieve placement in the most family-like setting available and in close proximity to the natural parents' home, consistent with the best interests of the child. Either a court or a panel of the state child welfare agency (at least one of whom is not responsible for the case) must review the plan at least every six months to determine the continued appropriateness of the placement, the extent of compliance with the plan, the progress towards eliminating the need for foster care, and the likely date by which the child may be returned to the home or placed for adoption or legal guardianship.

The courts have not hesitated to enforce the terms of the Act and the laws that preceded it. In *Lynch v. Dukakis* (1983), the United States Court of Appeals for the region that includes Massachusetts approved a preliminary injunction, that is, a court order to last until the final decision in the case, requiring that Massachusetts correct violations of the law that has now been replaced by the Adoption Assistance and Child Welfare Act, and that it conform to the law's requirements in providing case plans, furnishing services under the plans, and periodically reviewing the plans. Several foster children brought the case as a class action against the governor and other state officials.

Without disputing the *Lynch* decision, the United States Court of Appeals for the region that includes Ohio ruled in *Lesher v. Lavrich* (1986) that violations of the services requirements of the Adoption Assistance and Child Welfare Act do not entitle natural parents to sue to nullify a previous judgment of neglect and dependency and to obtain damages from state officials. It distinguished the classwide injunctive relief awarded in the *Lynch* case from damages relief in an individual case.

The *Lesher* decision, however, ignores the terms of a different federal statute providing an avenue of relief for violations of federal law (Civil Rights Act of 1871), which permits individual claims for damages against public officials, subject to various defenses such as good faith and sovereign immunity (*Maine v. Thiboutot*, 1980). Therefore, federal courts for other regions may decline to follow this precedent. At the minimum, foster children may enforce the Adoption Assistance and Child Welfare Act through individual hearings or class action lawsuits. This interpretation is confirmed by the Supreme Court's approval of the entry of a class action injunction against the State of Illinois for refusing to permit some persons to qualify as foster parents, in violation of a predecessor act (*Miller v. Youakim*, 1979).

In another context, one that involved neither a class action for an injunction nor an individual action for damages, the Delaware courts have barred the termination of parental rights because the state violated the Act in failing to provide services to facilitate reunification of the child with the natural parent (*In re Burns*, 1986; *Division of Child Protective Services v. Doran*, 1987). These cases demonstrate the effectiveness of a defensive use of the Act's provisions.

MEDICAL CARE

Children in foster care qualify for Medicaid (Social Security Act, Title XIX, 1935) on the basis of categorical eligibility under the Aid to Families with Dependent Children program (Adoption Assistance and Child Welfare Act, 1980). Medically complex children may also be categorically eligible on the basis of disability. Because of inadequate and slow reimbursement of medical providers by state Medicaid agencies, some providers are reluctant to accept Medicaid patients. Legal means to attack that problem include suits against providers on analogy to cases in which courts have found either negligence in transferring unstable patients who lack insurance coverage (*Brownsville Medical Center v. Garcia*, 1985), or violations of state emergency treatment statutes in refusing to render emergency aid (*Gonzalez v. United States*, 1985).

Beyond the availability of service providers, another problem with Medicaid is that the state medicaid plan may not cover all the treatment that a medically complex child needs. An alternative source of publicly funded care is state Crippled Children's Services (Social Security Act, Title V, 1935). That program provides medical, surgical, corrective, and other services, and funding for the necessary general care and facilities to provide those services, for children with special health care needs. In order to control expenditures, states commonly limit the children they serve by diagnosis. Snelling (1987) states that the inclusions and exclusions are based not on severity of condition or need for services, but on state administrators' capriciousness.

Snelling argues that the state programs' irrational exclusions from coverage violate section 504 of the federal Rehabilitation Act (1973), which forbids discrimination by federal grantees (in this instance, the states) against any otherwise qualified individual whose physical or mental impairments substantially limit one or more of the individual's major life activities. He distinguishes the exclusion of children by diagnosis in Crippled Children's programs from neutral caps on levels of services in Medicaid programs. The Supreme Court has found that the latter do not violate section 504 (*Alexander v. Choate*, 1985).

Because the Supreme Court has approved relief in lawsuits by handicapped persons against federal grantees who have discriminated against
them (*Consolidated Rail Corp. v. Darrone*, 1984), medically complex
children should be able to challenge exclusion from the Crippled
Children's programs in court. If funding shortages still require states
to impose limits on participation in the program, the courts might
force the states to impose more rational criteria, such as low income
status, severity of condition, or absence of duplication of services
through other programs. Medically complex foster children would
benefit most from Crippled Children's Services programs that would
provide medical services not available from Medicaid.

EDUCATIONAL SERVICES

Many medically complex children require special education in order
to get the most out of attending school. Others require no specialized
services, but may encounter resistance in their efforts to enroll in
regular classes. Much has been written about general legal issues in
special education (Weber, 1988; Weiner & Hume, 1987). With regard
to medically complex children in foster care, four specific categories
of information seem the most useful: procedures for identification
and placement of children; surrogate parent issues; rights pertaining
to placement in the least restrictive alternative; and the right of children with chronic infectious diseases to attend school.

Identification and Placement

The federal Education for All Handicapped Children Act (1975),
sometimes referred to as Public Law 94-142, requires states to provide
for the location, identification and evaluation of handicapped children
from birth. In most states, handicapped children have the right to
attend free, appropriate, public school from age three to graduation
from high school or age twenty-one. States will soon have in place
programs to serve handicapped children from birth to age three.

Upon a child's application or referral for special education, the
public school district must evaluate the child promptly, hold a meeting
with the child's parents or guardian to devise and individualized education program, and then place the child pursuant to that program.
Placement options must cover the full spectrum of learning environ-

ments, from attendance in regular classes with supplementary aids such as mechanical or audiovisual devices to enrollment at a residential school. Every year, the school district must review the placement and modify the program so that it remains appropriate. If the parents or guardian disagree with the program or placement, they may request a due process hearing from the superintendent of the school district. The child will remain in the existing placement until the completion of all hearings, appeals, and court review proceedings, unless the parents and the school agree otherwise. More details on the procedural framework of special education law are available elsewhere (Weber, 1988).

Public schools cannot summarily expel or suspend handicapped students. In *Honig v. Doe* (1988), the Supreme Court held that the Education for the Handicapped Act forbids public schools from suspending a handicapped child for more than ten days without affording the parents a right to a special education due process hearing. If the parents or guardian request the hearing, the child must remain in the existing placement pending the outcome of all proceedings, unless the school obtains an emergency order from a court.

Foster children are typically wards of the state. Since their natural parents are absent and their guardian, the state, may have interests that conflict with their need for potentially costly special education services, the law requires that surrogate parents be appointed to represent the child in all matters having to do with identification, evaluation, placement and provision of special education to the child (Code of Federal Regulations, Title 34, § 300.514, 1990). States must devise programs to select persons whose interests do not conflict with those of the child and to provide them with adequate knowledge and skills to represent the child. Foster parents are not automatically surrogate parents. They must be selected, agree to accept the responsibility, receive the necessary training, and be free of conflicting interests. The law bars employees of the child welfare agency and any other public agency that is involved in the education or care of the child from being the child's surrogate parent.

Least Restrictive Environment

Federal regulations enforcing the Education for All Handicapped Children Act provide (Code of Federal Regulations, Title 34. §550(b), 1990):

Each public agency shall insure:

(1) That to the maximum extent appropriate, handicapped children, including children in public or private institutions or other care facilities, are educated with children who are not handicapped, and

(2) That special classes, separate schooling or other removal of handicapped children from the regular educational environment occurs only when the nature or severity of the handicap is such that education in regular classes with the use of supplementary aids and services cannot be achieved satisfactorily.

This provision is sometimes referred to as the "mainstreaming" requirement. But as the language indicates, mainstreaming is not a negative command. There is no prohibition as such against placement in restrictive environments. It is instead a positive one: the Act mandates the school system to provide all the services that the child will need to succeed in the least restrictive environment possible. Those services need not be strictly educational. They may include such things as school health services, psychological services, group and individual counseling, audiology and anything else that assists a child to benefit from special education.

Cases support this positive interpretation of the mainstreaming requirement. In *Irving Independent School District v. Tatro* (1984), the Supreme Court held that a school had to supply clean intermittent catheterization for a student with a neurogenic bladder to permit her to attend school with other, nonhandicapped children. In an Illinois administrative review of a due process hearing decision, the State Board of Education ruled that a school district had to enroll a ventilator-dependent quadriplegic student in a public school class and provide him with the appliances and emergency medical backup to make the placement safe in the event of a mishap with his equipment (Case No. SE-27-84, 1984). A similar case is *Department of Education v. Katherine D.* (1984), a decision by the federal Court of Appeals for the region that includes Hawaii.

Chronic Infectious Disease

A final issue of concern to those assisting medically complex foster children in school matters is exclusion from school on the ground of chronic infectious disease. In the wake of the national epidemic of

Acquired Immune Deficiency Syndrome ("AIDS"), state education agencies have adopted chronic infectious disease policies. Those typically permit students with chronic infectious diseases to attend school without restriction except for circumstances where their behavior or other factors cause a significant risk of serious illness to others (Illinois State Board of Education and Illinois Department of Public Health, 1986).

Still, on numerous occasions school authorities have tried to exclude children who test positive for the human immunodeficiency virus ("HIV") antibody from public school. Absent extraordinary conditions, however, HIV-positive children should be able to attend classes without restriction, on the basis of section 504 of the Rehabilitation Act of 1973 and the Education for All Handicapped Children Act. Cases have proliferated on the topic of AIDS and the schools (Annotation, 1988; Rothstein, 1988), but the leading cases uphold the right of HIV-positive children to be treated the same as all other children.

Students who test positive for the HIV antibody are persons otherwise qualified to attend school whose major life activities are limited by a physical impairment. In *Thomas v. Atascadero Unified School District* (1987) a federal court in California issued a preliminary and then a permanent injunction forbidding a school district from excluding an HIV-positive student from his normal kindergarten class. The child had bitten a classmate during a skirmish. A psychologist, although unable to predict if the child would bite again, concluded that he would continue to act aggressively due to his low maturity level. The school argued for home tutoring for the child on the basis of federal guidelines which mention the potential risk of transmitting the AIDS virus through biting.

The court found the child's major life activities significantly impaired and therefore found him "handicapped" under the Rehabilitation Act. Further, the court concluded that the child was "otherwise qualified" to attend unrestricted classes, because treating physicians indicated there was no medical reason why he could not attend normal classes. The court also stressed the absence of any medical evidence that AIDS can be transmitted through human biting. The court concluded that the school had failed to comply with Rehabilitation Act regulations requiring that students who are handicapped be placed in the least restrictive environment.

Similarly, in *District 27 Community School Board v. Board of Education* (1986), a New York court rejected a school district's request for an order prohibiting an unidentified student with AIDS from attending New York City Public Schools. The district said that York City's Health Code excluded HIV-positive children from the public schools. The court held that section 504 of the Rehabilitation Act applies to those children. The court emphasized that the majority of testifying physicians stated that the risk of the AIDS being transmitted in the classroom is minimal at worst.

The court in *Ray v. School District* (1987), a federal case in Florida, imposed a preliminary injunction on a school system which tried to exclude three HIV-positive children from regular classes and force them to receive home instruction or attend a segregated classroom. The students had contracted AIDS infection through contaminated blood transfusions. The court noted the conclusions of a psychologist who had evaluated the children and found they would be irreparably harmed if they continued to be excluded from a normal classroom environment. The court also stated that the clear weight of medical testimony was that the children posed no foreseeable harm to other children, and therefore the public interest in protecting the educational rights and mental health of the HIV positive children outweighed any interest in protecting public health and safety. The court relied upon the Rehabilitation Act in concluding that the children were likely to win on the merits of the case and thus were entitled to a preliminary injunction.

In *Martinez v. School Board* (1988), the federal Court of Appeals for the region that includes Florida reversed the decision of a lower court, which had approved placing a six year-old mentally handicapped child who was HIV-positive in isolation within a classroom. The child was incontinent and drooled continually. The court rejected the idea that the remote, theoretical possibility of transmission of the disease justified the harm that the isolation would cause her.

Firm precedent and clear reasoning support the contention that HIV-positive children are "handicapped" under Section 504 of the Rehabilitation Act. If they are "otherwise qualified," they cannot be denied access to an unrestricted classroom. The interpretation of the Rehabilitation Act in the AIDS cases is consistent with the latest interpretation of the Act by the Supreme Court, in which it found that the Act covered a school teacher with tuberculosis and held that a court considering a suit challenging her dismissal should have considered whether she was otherwise qualified for her job (*School Board v. Arline*, 1987).

LEGAL ADVOCACY IN FOSTER CARE

HIV-positive students may also be protected by the Education for All Handicapped Children Act. They may use the Act to assert the right to a free, appropriate public education in the least restrictive environment. If the school authorities exclude them from school, they may invoke the provision of the law that keeps them in their existing placement or in regular classes if they have no existing special education placement. But the Act's definition of handicapped is that the student is so impaired as to be in need of special education; if all the student needs is to be in regular school, the Act will not apply. Moreover, in some cases, courts have found that HIV-positive students are not covered under the Act, reasoning further that because the students were not covered, they did not need to go through a due process hearing and otherwise exhaust administrative remedies before challenging their exclusion from school in court under section 504 (*Robertson v. Granite City Community Unit School District No. 9*, 1988; *Doe v. Belleville Public School District No. 118*, 1987). Resort to section 504 under that reasoning is likely to be unnecessary, however, in light of the Supreme Court's recent decision *Honig v. Doe* (1988), which affirmed that administrative remedies need not be exhausted if futile or inadequate, especially under "exigent circumstances," and which approved the entry of relief in a case where a student sued directly in court when he was excluded from school in violation of the provision requiring students to be kept in existing placements pending due process and appeal proceedings.

CONCLUSION

When a health or social work professional works to obtain public services for medically complex foster children, the professional must deal with bureaucracies that may not respond promptly or appropriately to the children's needs. Nevertheless, the programs the bureaucracies administer have legal underpinnings, and legal means exist to force the bureaucracies to give the children the services that are due them.

This chapter identifies the leading programs and the rights of children to services under the programs. Of course, variations in programs exist from state to state, and even when the entitlements are uniform, informal practices may vary. Informal practices of the public agencies provide opportunities for advocacy short of obtaining legal assistance and filing a hearing request or lawsuit. Local and statewide self-help organizations concentrating on rights of disabled persons provide crucial information and support for professionals engaging in informal advocacy efforts. Advocates for children with medically complex conditions will find their legal information put to its most effective use when they work with others in those organizations.

REFERENCES

Adoption Assistance and Child Welfare Act of 1980, 42 U.S.C. §§ 670, et seq. (1988).

Alexander v. Choate, 469 U.S. 287 (1985).

American Bar Association. (1983). *Model rules of professional conduct*. Chicago: Author.

Annotation. (1988). AIDS infection as affecting right to attend public school. *American Law Reports 4th, 60*, 15–35.

Brownsville Medical Center v. Garcia, 704 S.W.2d 68 (Tex. Ct. App. 1985).

Case No. SE-27-84, 1984–85 Educ. Handicapped L. Rep. 506: 103 (Ill. State Bd. of Educ. 1984).

Civil Rights Act of 1871, § 1, 42 U.S.C. § 1983 (1988).

Code of Federal Regulations, Title 34, §§ 300.514, 300.550(b) (1990).

Code of Federal Regulations, Title 45, §§ 1355.30(k), 1356.21(g)(1) (1989).

Consolidated Rail Corp. v. Darrone, 465 U.S. 624 (1984).

Department of Education v. Katherine D, 727 F.2d 809 (9th Cir. 1984), *cert. denied*, 471 U.S. 1117 (1985).

District 27 Community School Board v. Board of Education, 130 Misc. 2d 398, 502 N.Y.S.2d 325 (1986).

Division of Protective Servs. v. Doran, 529 A.2d 765 (Del. Fam. Ct. 1987).

Doe v. Belleville Public School Dist. No. 118, 672 F. Supp. 342 (S.D. Ill. 1987).

Education for All Handicapped Children Act of 1975, Public Law 94-142 (1975), 20 U.S.C. §§ 1400, et seq. (1988), as amended by Pub. L. 101-476, 104 Stat. 1103 (1990).

Gonzalez v. United States, 600 F. Supp. 1390 (W.D. Tex. 1985).

Hardin, M. (Ed.). (1983). *Foster children in the courts*. Boston: Butterworth.

Honig v. Doe, 484 U.S. 305 (1988).

Horowitz, R., Hardin, R., & Bulkley, J. (1989). *The rights of foster parents*. Washington, D.C.: American Bar Association.

Illinois Administrative Code, Title 89, § 359.4 (1988).

Illinois State Board of Education & Illinois Department of Public Health. (1986). *Management of chronic infectious diseases in school children*. Springfield, Ill.: State of Illinois.

In re Burns, 519 A.2d 638 (Del. 1986).

Irving Independent School District v. Tatro, 466 U.S. 923 (1984).

Lesher v. Lavrich, 784 F.2d 193 (6th Cir. 1986).

Lynch v. Dukakis, 719 F.2d 504 (1st Cir. 1983).

Maine v. Thiboutot, 448 U.S. 1 (1980).

Martinez v. School Board, 861 F.2d 1502 (11th Cir. 1988).

Miller v. Youakim, 440 U.S. 125 (1979).

Ray v. School District, 666 F. Supp. 1524 (M.D. Fla. 1987).

Rehabilitation Act of 1973, § 504, 29 U.S.C. § 794 (1988).

Robertson v. Granite City Community Unit School Dist. No. 9, 684 F. Supp. 1002 (S.D. Ill. 1988).

Rothstein, L. (1988). Children with AIDS: A need for a clear policy and procedure for public education, *Nova Law Review*. *12*, 1259–1289.

School Board v. Arline, 480 U.S. 273 (1987).

Snelling, P. (1987). Discrimination against children with special health care needs: Title V Crippled Children's Services programs and section 504 of the Rehabilitation Act of 1973, *Loyola University Law Journal*, *18*, 995–1009.

Social Security Act of 1935, Title V, 42 U.S.C. §§ 701, et seq., Title XIX, 42 U.S.C. §§ 1396, et seq., Title XX, 42 U.S.C. §§ 1397, et seq. (1988).

Thomas v. Atascadero Unified School District, 662 F. Supp. 376 (C.D. Cal. 1987).

Weber, M. (1988). Special education of handicapped children. In L. Foster (Ed.), *The Illinois Mental Health Professional's Law Handbook* (pp. 116–122). Chicago: The Editorial Committee.

Weiner, R. & Hume, M. (1987). *. . . And Education for All*. Alexandria, VA: Capitol Publications.

CHAPTER 16

ETHICAL ASPECTS OF PEDIATRIC HOME CARE

JOHN LANTOS
ARTHUR F. KOHRMAN

INTRODUCTION

Physicians, parents, nurses, administrators and politicians have recently changed their attitudes about pediatric home care for technology-dependent children. They have embraced the idea that chronically ill children can and should receive care at home rather than in hospitals, even if they have requirements for extensive and intensive high-technology care.

These changes were partly driven by the formidable possibilities of our new technologies, which allow many children to survive who would have died only a few years ago. Some of these children can only survive with a level of support equivalent to that available in intensive care units. Many of them, given that level of support, have the promise of significant intellectual development and functional capability. In response to the plight of these children, we have learned to build sophisticated intensive care units in the home, and to provide almost all of the sub-speciality and support functions and therapies found in the modern hospital. We have also learned that parents and other lay persons can be trained to do many of the instrumental tasks traditionally performed by medical care technologists and therapists in the hospital setting.

In addition to technological changes, psychological and philosophical factors have spurred changes in attitudes. Hospitals are not ideal places for children to grow and develop normally. The move to care at home is, in many cases, psychologically beneficial for the child.

Another important factor driving the changes in attitudes and practices has been a change in health care financing and the utilization of pediatric hospitals. There is a shortage of pediatric intensive care beds in the tertiary centers. At the same time, there is a shortage of beds for long-term care and a dearth of funds to pay for such care in inpatient settings. Pressures for cost-containment, both from payers and from the imperatives of prudent hospital management, lead to incentives for the development of alternative delivery systems. The driving forces here do not, of course, necessarily coincide with the best interests of the patient, and may, in fact, represent some of the least admirable aspects of the contemporary health care system. However, when a change seemingly enhances both the best interest of the patients and appears to meet the demands of cost containment, it may become irresistible in the present climate.

These forces and attitudes represent a combination of the humane, the economic, the organizational and the political. For each decision to provide medical care for a child at home, a mixture of these and other motives exists. One of the goals of the present chapter is to stimulate identification and analysis of the social forces and individual motives which enter into each decision to send a medically complex child home. We will also raise some issues which have become apparent as consequences of our decisions to send technology-dependent children home have unfolded over the last several years (Kohrman, 1984). To do this, we will first survey the range of home health care. We will then discuss generally some of the ethical issues that arise. Finally, we will focus on home ventilator therapy to highlight the ethical dilemmas that arise in pediatric home care.

THE RANGE OF HOME HEALTH CARE

Home health care in pediatrics begins with prenatal care. Pregnant women make certain lifestyle changes, take medicines, and comply with prenatal care visit schedules as part of their responsibility to their child. Assistance in childbirth is a form of health care that was once predominantly provided in the home. The move from home to hospital was brought about because of perceived benefits to both mothers and babies. In recent years, some have argued that these benefits may have been overestimated, or that they only apply to sub-populations with high risk factors (Hoff & Schneiderman, 1985).

The home care of routine transient childhood illnesses is seen as a parental obligation. Parents who want to hospitalize their child for fever, diarrhea or other self-limited illnesses are not permitted to do so. On the other hand, parents are legally required to bring their child for medical care if their children are ill. Failure in this responsibility is seen as neglect or even as child abuse (Bross, 1982). Parents are expected to show good judgement in making the decision to seek medical evaluation, and to trust physicians' judgement regarding decisions to care for their children at home or in the hospital.

In recent years, the scope of home health care has widened to include the sophisticated treatment regimens prescribed for asthma, cystic fibrosis (McDonald, 1981), diabetes mellitus (Hopper, Miller, Birge, & Swift, 1984), and other chronic conditions. Children may receive intravenous antibiotics (Rehm & Weinstein, 1983), hyperalimentation (Dahlstrom, Strandvik, Kapple & Ament, 1985), oxygen, (Donn, 1982) renal dialysis, and even mechanical ventilation at home (Burr, Guyer, & Todres, 1983). The complete range of home health care services also includes end-of-life care for children with terminal disease. Hospice programs have begun to develop to provide services and assistance to parents who wish to have their children at home at the time of death (Edwardson, 1985).

With the development of more complex life-support systems that can be placed in the home, we must ask whether there are limits to the burdens that parents must shoulder in providing for their children's care. The criteria of judging parents as acceptable if they provide health care or neglectful if they do not break down in the face of technologies like home mechanical ventilation, home dialysis, or home parenteral nutritional therapy. At these points along the spectrum of home health care, there is the possibility for legitimate disagreement between parents and physicians about the risks and benefits of home versus hospital care, and about the boundaries of legitimate authority for deciding between options. In these areas, there may be a middle ground, in which parents can elect not to become primary health care providers, but still maintain moral authority over their children's care. By forcing us to make the distinctions that will define this middle ground, the "new" home health care serves as a lens through which our traditional conceptions of parental responsibility can be examined.

ETHICAL ISSUES IN HOME HEALTH CARE

The ethical issues around pediatric home care can be conceptualized around two major axes: first, the nature of parental participation in decision-making for taking and keeping the child home; and second, the clarification of the medical professionals' values and institutional traditions and the assumptions and behaviors that grow from them. Central to consideration of the latter is the definition of 'acceptable' risk and the distribution of responsibility between professionals and parents forced by moving the focus of care to the home.

The decision to discharge hospitalized children is legally, traditionally and instrumentally the physician's decision. Other health-care professionals are also very involved in the decision making process, and particularly in the implementation of the discharge to home. Thus, the issues to be raised must be confronted by all who participate, regardless of their professional designation; nonetheless, this discussion will focus on physician-led decision making.

Choosing possible candidates for home discharge is possibly the most important decision of all. It initiates and foreordains the subsequent decisions, choices and actions. Here, indeed, the most important ethical issue may appear: is the question of home discharge initiated by the parents (and, if possible, the child) or is it posed by the professionals? In either case, is a choice made with the full range of options evident to the family, or is it presented to or perceived by the family as a mandate rather than a choice? If the dialogue is professionally initiated and driven, what are the motives for the selection of a particular patient? Is it because of a bed shortage or inadequate payment available for needed services? Does the hospital environment make it impossible for parents to hesitate, or to refuse responsibilities of home care without guilt? Is a parental choice for home care driven by social or extended family pressures to demonstrate "good" parenting? Less evident are decisions not to offer home-care as an option because of judgments about the abilities of the caretakers. Such judgments are necessary, but should not be made on the basis of untested and possibly prejudicial assumptions based on a family's socioeconomic status or structure.

Physicians and nurses carry the psychological and legal burdens of responsibility for "bad" outcomes. Moving a technology-dependent child out of the hospital to the home creates several strains on these deeply-felt obligations. First, reordering of what are 'good' and what are 'bad' outcomes may be necessary; even survival, under some circumstances of continuous intensive, isolated, uncomfortable existence may not always be the most important outcome. The restoration of the family, if only for a clearly shortened duration, may take precedence over the nuances of "ideal" care (as defined at that time and in that place—both somewhat slippery standards). Second, participation of families and children in truly shared decision-making may result in a hierarchy of choices different from that of the professionals acting from their traditional imperatives. Third, once a child is home, professionals no longer directly participate in the daily care of the patient. They may still feel responsible, however, and the changing ratio of responsibility and control may cause professionals intolerable anxiety.

In order to more concretely illustrate these dilemmas, we will discuss the ethical issues in home health care by focusing on home ventilator therapy. Although this therapy is at one end of the spectrum of the range of services that can be classified as 'home health care,' it is paradigmatic for the type of considerations that must be kept in mind as we move from a hospital environment to a home environment.

HOME VENTILATOR CARE: A PARADIGM

History of Home Ventilator Care

Home ventilator therapy is perhaps the most controversial of home therapies. Ventilator therapy is traditionally thought of as an intensive care unit (ICU) therapy. Home ventilator care is labor-intensive, and the consequences of a failure of either technical or human systems often can be the immediate death of the child. Yet, in spite of these formidable considerations, many children who require ventilators do not require any other hospital care. They and/or their parents may feel that continued confinement to the ICU constitutes an undesirable burden.

Home ventilator care developed as a response to political pressure from British polio patients who felt that they should be provided with the services necessary to enable them to leave their hospitals (Goldberg, 1984). Similar programs were developed in France and the United States. Home ventilator care for children had been attempted, on a sporadic basis, since at least 1965 in the United States (Frates, Splaingard, Smith & Harrison, 1985).

The impetus to develop home ventilator programs increased in 1981 when President Reagan announced that eligibility rules for federal payment would be waived to allow a ventilator-dependent child, Katie Beckett, to return home. Shortly afterward, Surgeon General C. Everett Koop convened a national conference to discuss the care of the ventilator-dependent child (Kohrman, 1984).

Safety and Efficacy of Pediatric Home Ventilator Care

The development of programs for home ventilation preceeded evaluation of the safety and effectiveness of this innovative therapeutic
modality. Only now is research being done on the effectiveness of
home-based ventilator care for children. It has focused on three areas—
(1) the safety of home ventilator as compared to hospital treatment;
(2) the cost of home ventilation; and, most recently, (3) the social
impact of home versus hospital therapy, both for children and for
their families.

The data are complex. Randomized controlled trials of home ventilator therapy are not feasible. The reported series are retrospective
studies of carefully selected patients and families who met very narrow
medical and social criteria. Even in these groups, mortality statistics
vary widely. Goldberg, Faure and Vaughn (1984) followed 18 children
for up to 6 years, and reported only 1 death (6% mortality). Frates,
Splaingard, Smith and Harrison (1985) followed 54 children for up
to 20 years. Seventeen (32%) children died, and 3 of those deaths
resulted from accidental ventilator disconnection. One year survival
in that study was 84% and five year survival 65%. Burr et al. (1983)
followed 6 children for up to 7 years at home. None of these children
died, but one was described as "deteriorating."

Only one series included data on both hospital and home care of
infants with chronic respiratory failure. Schriener, Downes and Kettrick (1987) described 101 infants who required mechanical ventilation
for more than 28 days in the first year of life. Overall mortality was
30%, with half of the deaths occurring in the 12 months following
diagnosis of chronic respiratory failure. Six of the 30 deaths were
caused by airway related accidents (accidental decannulation, unrec-
ognized obstruction of tracheostomy tube, or ventilator disconnection), and 5 of these accidental deaths occurred at home. In 3 of
these 5, the patient was no longer on mechanical ventilation at the
time of death.

These studies show that, although home ventilation can be safe
and effective for some children, it is a risky form of therapy. They
do not tell whether it is as safe as ventilation in the hospital. In order
to answer this question, it would be necessary to have statistics on
ventilator dependent children with comparable medical problems cared
for in ICUs, skilled nursing units, and homes. These data do not
exist.

Cost-effectiveness of Home Ventilator Care

Similar uncertainty exists in evaluating the cost-effectiveness of home ventilator therapy. Initially, it was felt that home ventilator therapy would be much less expensive than hospital therapy, as other home therapies have proved to be. Early reports confirmed this, showing that home care costs were 50 to 95% lower than hospital costs (Goldberg, Faure & Vaughn, 1984). More recent data has tempered some of the initial optimism. In the original reports, the *costs* of home care were compared to the *charges* for ICU care. ICU charges may be higher than actual costs. Home care costs tend to be underestimated because they ignore both lost income by a parent who needs to stop work in order to be a full time caretaker and the value of the parent's time in providing care. When children at home are cared for on a 24-hour basis by registered nurses, the cost of home care approaches the cost of hospital care for the same child (Aday, Aitken, Wegener & Dranove, 1988). In addition, the success of home ventilator care has led to the development of skilled nursing units, where costs are much lower than in ICUs. No reports have yet compared costs of either home or hospital care with costs in a skilled nursing facility or in a transitional-care setting.

Assessments of quality of life for patients at home have been attempted, but have suffered from both the idiosyncracies of the patient selection process and the lack of comparable control groups. Goldberg et al. (1984) reports that "children with documented developmental delay in the hospital have demonstrated a remarkable rate of progress at home . . . The added responsibilities of home care to the families have been a minor burden . . ." Burr et al. (1983), on the other hand, acknowledges that most of the children they studied had not received developmental assessments to clarify their educational and social needs. Many had difficulty finding educational programs that could handle ventilator dependent children. Frates et al. (1984) reports that 28% of their children attend regular school and 23% attend special school. Eleven percent of the families in Frates' study either refused to take their children home, or transferred them to nursing homes after some years of caring for them at home.

The psychosocial benefits of home care would seem to be potentially large, but in any given situation are influenced by many variables, including parental motivation, community support, and economic resources. The contribution of each of these factors, and the role of other non-elucidated factors, remains unknown. Until more complete data are available, there is a strong ethical imperative to reveal all the uncertainties inherent in the home care of medically-dependent children to parents or others contemplating such care. In addition, these uncertainties must be honestly faced by the professionals as they evaluate and select candidates for home care.

PROFESSIONAL RESPONSIBILITY: DECISION MAKING UNDER CONDITIONS OF UNCERTAINTY

The physician who cares for a ventilator-dependent child must make decisions surrounded by considerable uncertainty. It is difficult to interpret ethical principles which should guide such decisionmaking. It is axiomatic, for example, that treatment should only be provided if it is medically efficacious; however, there is considerable uncertainty about the efficacy of home ventilator therapy compared to hospital-based treatment.

Physicians might try to minimize the uncertainty by creating generalizations from existing knowledge. Using that approach, the data already gathered on the medical efficacy, psychosocial advantages, and cost-effectiveness of home health care might be interpreted as an unqualified mandate to shift as much ventilator care as possible from hospital to home settings. This would be a mistake. The existing data are ambiguous, both in regard to the overall efficacy of home care versus hospital care, and with regard to the effect of patient selection criteria on outcome. A critical assessment of the available data suggest that they create more questions than they answer.

One positive way to view these results is that they ethically justify further research. In order to conduct ethical research, there should be genuine uncertainty about the benefits of an innovative therapy, as compared to a standard therapy (Freedman, 1987). This situation now exists with regard to home ventilator therapy. Research projects should try to answer the questions which have been raised.

While research should go on, the clinical circumstances in which decisions about home and hospital care must be made may not be conducive to the type of studies which might answer the most important questions. Randomization would be difficult to achieve, even within carefully designed selection criteria, because any parents who really wanted to take their child home would not sign up for a study in which one arm of the study entailed continued hospitalization. On the other hand, requiring someone to take their child home who was unwilling to do so may constitute experimentation without the consent of the subject. The desire to gather good data conflicts with the imperative to respect patients' interests.

Uncertainty, then, is not a temporary state that will give way to knowledged, but an inherent characteristic of clinical decision making for ventilator-dependent children. Uncertainty changes the role of the physician from one who determines which course is in the child's best interest to one who must enter into the process of education and negotiation with a family, in order to help the family decide on a course of action.

In these circumstances, physician responsibility has at least two meanings—responsiveness to patient needs, and responsibility for outcomes, good and bad. The two meanings often conflict, and physicians have a tendency to fall back on the latter concept of responsibility as the one which ethically preempts the former. This fall back leads to decisions which maximize physician control over process, in order to absolutely minimize bad sequelae. The tendency to keep children in the hospital because the risks at home are higher results from this conceptualization of responsibility.

The other construction of professional responsibility resembles more the traditional parental conceptions of responsibility. Parents are always faced with decisions about how much it is justifiable to limit their children's risky behaviors. Known health and safety benefits must be balanced against the psychosocial needs of children to take responsibility for themselves and to learn how to make their way in the world. Viewed in this way, the parent/child negotiation can be seen as analogous to the negotiation that goes on between physician and parent. The physician may have a deeper understanding of the exact nature of the risks of home care, but the parent knows the family's needs and strengths. Physician authority and stature can preempt any opportunity for a family to come to know itself or to grow; however, properly used, it can encourage families to consider all available options.

There exists, then, a spectrum of physician responsibility. Where to place oneself on that spectrum depends on the assessments of the true risk of any course of action. In making this assessment, physicians need to remember that the goal is not the elimination of risk but the reasonable reduction of risk.

SELECTION OF CANDIDATES FOR HOME CARE

All hospital programs which prepare children and families for discharge to home care have established more or less restrictive and detailed criteria of physiologic stability of the child, for education of the caretakers and for preparation of the receiving environment (Frates et al., 1985; Goldberg, 1984; Schreiner, Downes & Kettrick, 1987; Aday, Aitken, Wegener & Dranove, 1988). There are reasonable and generally accepted standards for such determination.

The criteria of adequacy for the family wanting to care for a medically complex child at home will vary with the needs of the child. For children with short or nonexistent periods of tolerance of equipment failure, it is reasonable to require that at least two competent caretakers be ordinarily available. For many chronically ill children cared for at home a single, responsible individual with access to other resources and help will suffice.

Parents must be willing to take a medically complex child home for care. Such a decision must be based on judgments that it is in the child's and family's best balanced interests. Other motivations—particularly economic or bureaucratic ones—which ignore or devalue those interests cannot ethically be allowed to dominate. In addition, experience shows that the family which has made a reluctant decision to care for their child at home under pressure, overt or implicit, from their extended family, their peers or their medical caregivers are at high risk of failure, especially if the demands of the child are complex. Indeed, it has been observed that, under conditions of extreme stress resulting from coerced choices for home care, the parents may become patently neglectful or even abusive of their disabled child (Sargent, 1983).

The training of the future caretakers of the child in the home or alternative setting must be well thought out, meticulous, extensive and intensive. Standards for knowledge and performance must be established and their mastery and competence ascertained before the child is discharged and periodically thereafter. The care of a medically complex child in the home is an extraordinary challenge, and inadequate preparation of the caretakers and the environment constitutes a serious professional breach.

In a similar vein, it is incumbent upon the professionals arranging for the discharge of the child to home care to be certain that not only are the necessary resources, personnel and equipment available at the time of discharge, but that they will be assured for the future. It is not ethically nor morally acceptable to discharge a child knowing that there are not funds or resources available for necessary and optimal care beyond a limited time. The obligation of the professionals in the discharging institution extends beyond its walls and beyond the immediate future; they must ascertain that another competent agency or system will assume responsibility for care, enforcement of care standards and advocacy for child and family if they themselves are not willing or prepared to do so.

CONCLUSIONS

The recent trend to care for medically complex and technology-dependent children in the home has created many ethical dilemmas and choices. In this area, the best interests of the child and family should be the guiding ethical principle. Because the care of a medically complex child in the home imposes significant changes in the responsibilities of family members, it may be necessary to construct a calculus of collective best interest to find an ethically satisfying position.

Traditional professional attitudes and behaviors in hospital-based care, which seek to minimize risk at any cost, must be changed to permit joint decision-making and acceptance of shared risk by the family of the child to be cared for at home. Professionals must not adhere to narrowly defined standards of acceptable risk. However, physicians and other medical personnel have the obligation to make certain that families understand the challenges and hazards of home care for medically complex children and to ensure that families are well-trained and confident in the details of the child's care before discharge. The decision to discharge a medically-complex child to home carries with it the obligation to assure that the caretakers are trained in all aspects of care of the child and know how to obtain emergency and supportive consultation. Similarly, all the fiscal and material resources needed for the child's extended care at home must be in place. To create and execute a care plan which is incomplete or inadequate in these regards is an ethical failure as well as an almost-certain functional failure.

More data about the efficacy and hazards of home care will resolve some of the present uncertainties, and clarify the related decisions. However, the ethical obligations of full disclosure, adequate preparation of the family and the possibility of renegotiation with dignity will remain. If these obligations are fulfilled, the sharing of risk with families of medically complex children becomes acceptable, and many children and their families will have their best interests served as the possibilities of pediatric home care unfold.

The limits of parental obligations to severely impaired or technology-dependent children are presently unclear. Professionals must not force parents, by implication or explicitly, to assume obligations for care which are clearly extraordinary or beyond their capabilities, or they will inevitably create great guilt or a sense of failure in the family members who decline to assume those obligations.

REFERENCES

Aday, L. A., Aitken, J. M., Wegener, D. H. & Dranove, D. (1988). Pediatric Home Care: Results of a national evaluation of programs for ventilator assisted children. Chicago: Pluribus Press.

Bross, D. (1982). Medical neglect. *Child Abuse and Neglect, 6,* 375–81.

Burr, B. H., Guyer, B. Todres, I. D., Abraham, B., & Chiodo, T. (1983). Home care for children on respirators. *New England Journal of Medicine, 309,* 1319–23.

Dahlstrom, K. A., Strandvik, B., Kapple, J., & Ament, M. E. (1985). Nutritional status in children receiving home parental nutrition. *Journal of Pediatrics, 107,* 219–24.

Donn, S. (1982). Cost effectiveness of home management of bronchopulmonary dysplasia. *Pediatrics, 70,* 330–1.

Edwardson, S. R. (1985). Physician acceptance of home care for terminally ill children. *Health Service Research, 20,* 83–100.

Frates, R. C., Splaingard, M. L., Smith, E. O., & Harrison, G. M. (1985). Outcome of home mechanical ventilation in children. *Journal of Pediatrics, 106,* 850–6.

Freedman, B. (1987). Equipoise and the ethics of clinical research. *New England Journal of Medicine, 317,* 141–145.

Goldberg, A. I. (1984). Home care services for the ventilator dependent person in England and France. *Proceedings of the Brook Lodge Invitational Symposium on the Ventilator-Dependent Child* (pp. 1–3). La Rabida Children's Hospital and The Upjohn Co.

Goldberg, A. I., Faure, E. A. M., Vaughn, C. J., Snorski, R., & Seleny, F. L. (1984). Home care for life supported persons: an approach to program development. *Journal of Pediatrics, 104,* 785–95.

Hoff, G. A. & Schneiderman, L. J. (1985). Having babies at home: Is it safe? Is it ethical? *Hastings Center Report, 15,* 19–27.

Hopper, S. V., Miller, J. P., Birge, C., & Swift, J. (1984). A randomized study of the impact of home health aides on diabetic control and utilization patterns. *American Journal of Public Health, 74*, 600–2.

Kohrman, A. (1984). Pediatric home care: A ten-point agenda for the future. In *Home Care for Children with Serious Handicapping Conditions* (pp. 98–105). Washington, DC: The Association for the Care of Children's Health.

McDonald, G. J. (1981). A home care program for children with chronic lung disease. *Nursing Clinics of North America, 16*, 259–73.

Rehm, S. J., & Weinstein, A. J. (1983). Home intravenous antibiotic therapy: a team approach. *Annals of Internal Medicine, 99*, 388–92.

Sargent, J. (1983). The sick child: Family complications. *Journal of Developmental Behavioral Pediatrics, 4*, 50–6.

Schreiner, M. S., Downes, J. J. & Kettrick, R. G. (1987). Chronic respiratory failure in infants with prolonged ventilator dependency. *Journal of the American Medical Association, 258*, 3398–3404.

CHAPTER 17

FINANCING CARE FOR MEDICALLY COMPLEX CHILDREN

STEVE A. FREEDMAN
LESLIE L. CLARKE

INTRODUCTION

Like all medical care, the delivery of health care services to medically complex children in the United States is determined by the systems that finance such care (Blendon, 1982). Moreover, health care financing mechanisms determine not only the type of medical services and how these services are delivered, but also who receives and who delivers the services (Select Panel for the Promotion of Child Health, 1981). Unfortunately, systems for providing families of medically complex children with financial assistance for needed services are very fragmented and largely inadequate. The conditions that befall and characterize medically complex children are extremely expensive and rarely anticipated, yet few public or private health insurance plans cover medical care for these children once the medical bills have exceeded policy limits or after the child has left the hospital. Moreover, recent trends have shown that this population and the costs of medical technology are continuing to grow. Consequently, assessment of current and alternative systems for the funding of care for medically complex children is an important step in the development of adequate systems of care. Attention to the following questions is essential: Who should pay for necessary medical care when the family cannot? How can care and/or financial assistance to this population be most equitably distributed? And how can cost-effective systems of transitional, home and school care be developed that maintain acceptable levels of quality? Indeed the ability of health care professionals and policy-makers to adequately address these questions will determine the future course of the health care delivery system.

The growth in the number of medically complex children and the shift in recent years from institutionalized care to home and community-based care for disabled and chronically ill children has placed additional emphasis on the import and timeliness of the issue of financing care. The following discussions are intended to provide a general framework for addressing the issues by appraising the current systems of care and financing and their effectiveness. Specifically, the purpose of this chapter is to critically assess current and proposed systems of public and private financing of services for medically complex children and to make recommendations for the development of policy and programs for the improvement of services.

Assessment of the adequacy of systems that pay for care, however, cannot occur without discussions of quality and appropriateness of care for these children. Recently the Task Force on Technology Dependent Children, a congressionally mandated committee of experts, presented an extensive report on the barriers to the provision of appropriate care for technology dependent children (Task Force, 1988). In this report the Task Force outlines a number of critical problems and barriers to appropriate care faced by these children and their families. The data and insights concerning these components of appropriate care are used as a template for this discussion. Our discussions, therefore, include assessment of the type and adequacy of services offered by each system as well as the financing of services in order to highlight the link between cost and quality. We discuss the costs of services and problems in service delivery in the context of appropriateness of services in order to emphasize the difficult questions policy makers and health professionals must face.

We begin our task by briefly describing the demographic and medical characteristics of the medically complex population and their families, with attention to issues that make this population financially vulnerable. Next, after reviewing the components of appropriate care outlined by the Task Force, the current systems of funding care for medically complex children are reviewed and assessed in light of their adequacy. We then review alternative (i.e., new or proposed) mechanisms of funding that are believed to improve on existing programs and better provide funding for the "appropriate" care recommended by the Task Force. We close by summarizing and recommending directions for future development of policies aimed at funding care for medically complex children.

MEDICALLY COMPLEX CHILDREN AND THEIR CARE

An estimated 10 to 15 percent of all children in the United States have a chronic health condition, with about 1 million of these having costly and disabling conditions (General Accounting Office, 1989). Data from the National Health Interview Survey (NHIS) show that over two million children suffer some degree of activity limitation due to their health or disability, of which about 95,000 have conditions interfering with school attendance (Newacheck, Budetti and Mc-Manus, 1984). Moreover, the size of the technology-dependent population, as a subgroup of the medically complex population is estimated at between 17,000 and 100,000 children (Office of Technology Assessment, 1987). This estimated range is a function of the varying definitions and levels of technology-dependence used and reflects the lack of hard data on this population. The population of children requiring ventilator assistance, nutritional, or other medical support, for example, is estimated at 2,300 to 17,000. The number of children requiring apnea monitoring, renal dialysis, or other device-associated care is between 37,800 and 81,000.

Despite the great need for more accurate data on the size and characteristics of the medically complex population, these data are not available. It is known, however, that this population continues to grow due to the increasing number of physically compromised and technology-dependent children who survive neonatal and general intensive technological medical care. For example, the increasing survival rates of very low birthweight infants due to technological interventions has resulted in increasing numbers of infants dependent on ventilators and intravenous feeding. While the benefits gained by the advancement of medical technology in the area of neonatology are significant, the attendant costs to the child, the family, and to society are considerable. Appropriate utilization of resources, as well as attention to improved access for all children to necessary medical care, are goals requiring constant monitoring and assessment.

The history of health care financing for medically complex children indicates growing public and legislative concern. Many legislative initiatives, however, have created a public system of finance characterized as "fragmented and capricious" due to poor interagency coordination, lack of program development, and/or funding concerns (Hobbs, Perrin & Ireys, 1985). State variations in Medicaid eligibility and coverage, for instance, leave many poor chronically ill children without medical care. And though over half of all children with major health problems are covered by private health insurance, many of these policies either do not cover the expenses associated with medically complex conditions, have high co-payments or deductibles, and/ or have maximum spending limits that are well below the costs of care for medically complex children (Task Force, 1988). Moreover, the population of children who have severe medical limitations is found to have lower rates of private insurance coverage than children without such medical limitations. According to the 1982 National Health Interview Survey, 53.8% of non-institutionalized children with severe limitations of activity, compared to 74.3% of children without any limitations have private health insurance (Office of Technology Assessment, 1987). This figure is consistent with other findings that indicate that the poor and those without medical insurance have poorer health (Butler, Winter, Singer & Wenger, 1985; Freedman, Klepper, Duncan & Bell, 1988). Consequently, the size of the population of children with considerable medical needs yet with inadequate or no health insurance coverage is increasing.

The Task Force On Technology-Dependent Children, established in 1986 to "identify barriers that prevent the provision of appropriate care in a home or community setting to meet the special needs of technology-dependent children" (Task Force, 1988), report three principles as guides to the adequacy of care for technology-dependent children. These principles include: 1) equitable access to appropriate services for all children; 2) family-centered, community-based, coordinated and comprehensive care systems; and 3) the rendering of services in the least restrictive environment (Task Force, 1988). These principles form the foundation upon which their other more specific recommendations rest. For example, they further recommend that the financing of appropriate care should include the following: 1) universal access; 2) cost-efficient care; 3) family financial responsibility; 4) family participation in care management; 5) creative delivery of services to facilitate habilitative capability of the child; 6) public-private third party cooperation; 7) assurance of high quality care; and 8) expansion of service capacity on the local level (Task Force, 1988). So, the development of program to serve and finance care for the medically complex must not only meet criteria of adequacy but they should also address problems of access, cost-containment, quality, family involvement and organizational cooperation. These goals present a substantial challenge to current systems of medical care provision and financing.

With appropriate planning and utilization of public and private sector support, the Task Force believes that these goals can be achieved with limited increase in federal expenditures. To do this, the private sector is viewed as the necessary payer of first resort, with the enhancement of federal and state policy and resources to improve health insurance benefits. Furthermore, improved coordination of existing medical services and financial resources, and the expansion of publicly-financed third-party reimbursement based on "family health-related out-of-pocket expenditures" (Task Force, 1988) are recommended. In addition, the identification and coordination of medical services locally, regionally and nationally would improve access as well as reduce the costly duplication of health care resources.

Another suggestion for cost-containment without service reduction is to improve the funding of home and community-based care. However, a paucity of adequate data exists on the cost-effectiveness of such care, with the exception of data from Medicaid waiver programs (Office of Technology Assessment, 1987). In addition to the difficulty in comparing home and hospital care and cost savings, the bias of most health insurance policies toward hospital care and away from non-institutional alternatives has prevented families from having the option of home care and society from weighing the differences. Moreover, most medical care funding mechanisms, such as third-party insurance policies, do not cover additional support needs of caring for medically complex children at home, such as nursing care, transportation, or respite care, rendering home care especially unaffordable.

Given this background, we next present the four components of appropriate care proposed by the Task Force as guides to the assessment and improvement of services for medically complex children. These components include: 1) Case Management; 2) Developmental/Educational Services; 3) Family Support; and 4) Respite Care. Each of these components of appropriate care are described below as they are relevant to a discussion of the adequacy of financing mechanisms.

COMPONENTS OF APPROPRIATE CARE

Case Management

Noted as the most important, case management is the first component of appropriate care described by the Task Force. In general, case management refers to any system that directs the flow of services and financing to a patient. The Task Force defines case management as "a goal-oriented process which promotes the effective and efficient organization and utilization of medical, social, educational and other resources to achieve or maintain the maximum potential of the child in the most appropriate, least restrictive environment." This includes systems that focus on cost-containment, benefits coordination, family support, and the monitoring of services. Moreover, case management is considered a "dynamic process with the child and family at its center, moving along a continuum of assessment, goal-setting, delivery of services, evaluation, and reassessment."

In this context the task force recommends an emphasis on "cost-avoidance" in goal-oriented case management as having the greatest potential for "assuring that the client receive necessary services without inappropriately utilizing costly resources" and for avoiding reinstitutionalization. The extent to which any levels of case management have been integrated into public or private programs, however, is not fully known. Although Congress has expressed a commitment to the development of case management services in Medicaid, Title V Program for Children with Special Health Needs, and The Education for the Handicapped Act Amendments of 1986 (Public Law 99-457), the widespread utilization of this approach to service delivery is still underdeveloped.

Developmental/Educational Services

The goals of developmental services in the provision of appropriate care are defined as, first, to foster the maximum social and educational development of medically complex children, and second, to mainstream them into community schools whenever possible (Office of Technology Assessment, 1987). The barriers to the achievement of these goals include, for example, reluctance of school systems to admit such children, a lack of federal and state guidelines on "where responsibility lies in the provision of and payment for services to a technology-dependent child in school," and a lack of attention to developmental needs during acute care hospitalization (Task Force, 1988).

To overcome these barriers, the task force recommends that Congress review existing school health procedures and develop guidelines to ensure care of technology-dependent children in schools. They also recommend the federal support to assist states in identifying and developing appropriate in-service training for all school personnel, and to clarify the coordination of benefits and financial relationships among the various federal programs for the support of health care services to technology-dependent children.

Family Support

Family support is defined as "services, resources, information, training and emotional support that enables a family to assume responsibility and provide care for a technology-dependent child in addition to meeting goals and accomplishing tasks of family life" (Task Force, 1988). A recent study, however, reports that community-based social support services are widely lacking (Walker, Palfrey, Butler & Singer, 1988). From their survey of families of functionally disabled children, these authors also conclude that until more attention is placed on making these services available, the goal of improved family-centered, community-based care children will not be achieved. A lack of a partnership between parents and professionals, and of support systems to aid parents in planning and providing appropriate care for their child are noted as major barriers to the expansion of family support services. To overcome these barriers, the Task Force (1987) recommends a wider acceptance of the family-centered and community-based approach to care, as well as the development of a parent-professional partnership and a comprehensive information network for families of these children.

Respite Care

Respite care is a service for the family that provides an alternate to or substitute for family caregiving responsibilities of their technology dependent child on a planned or unscheduled basis. It may take place in the home or other appropriate location. This service should be provided by individual(s) with qualifications appropriate to the provision of the child's care (Task Force, 1988). In addition, respite care is viewed as a necessary component in a continuum of appropriate care. Unfortunately, profound barriers to the access of respite care by families of medically complex children exist today. The major barrier to access to respite care services are first, that the services are simply not available, and second, where they are available, funding sources and aid to parents who wish to utilize the services are limited. A recent study reports that less than 15% of the families of children with Cerebral Palsy, Muscular Dystrophy and other illnesses surveyed said they had used any kind of respite care services in the previous year (Walker et al., 1988).

Recommendations for the expansion of respite care include: 1) the allocation of federal funds to develop national guidelines for respite care service, implementation, and development of volunteer networks; 2) the provision of incentives to insurance purchasers to include respite care in their benefit packages; and 3) to require respite care as a component of the individualized plan for technology-dependent children.

These recommendations for the improvement of the quality and comprehensiveness of care for medically complex children are important goals, but do not come without a cost. The questions of how to implement and pay for these services is central to the implementation of such recommendations. The next section reviews the major public, private and cooperative funding strategies for the care of medically complex children in the U.S. today.

CURRENT FINANCING STRATEGIES

Medical and health care services in the United States are funded through one of three major systems: the private, the public, or a combination of private and public systems. The private sector includes all third-party insurance providers which provide coverage to individual and groups, and private philanthropic organizations, such as the March of Dimes, which provide funding for services and research. While some private hospitals provide services to the indigent, this mechanism is not considered a viable private system of funding because the cost of such care is ultimately billed to existing private and public payers.

Public sector funding mechanisms include all federal and state-supported programs such as Medicare, Medicaid and the Title V Program for Children with Special Health Needs, which provide funding for medical care for a variety of populations including children, the elderly, disabled or poor, or disease-specific programs created and maintained through public funds.

Cooperative private and public mechanisms, the least common of the three funding sources, include programs supported jointly by government and private agencies. The cooperative arrangements of public and private organizations in the delivery of services previously provided by the government is an area of growing support despite on-going debates over the consequences of privatization. In light of the inadequacies of current systems of funding and delivery of care for the medically complex, the coordination of public and private systems has emerged as one of the more popular avenues of program development. In fact, the Task Force recommended a consortium of public and private agencies to administer the financing of services for medically complex children (described below).

The specific programs that currently provide support for the care of medically complex children within each of these systems are described below. In Table 17.1 we have summarized the private and public programs currently available, including their eligibility requirements, coverage provided, and state participation, as a synopsis of the discussions to follow (with the exclusion of public-private cooperative programs). After the review of current programs, we discuss alternative programs of financing and care.

Private Sector Funding Sources

The private sector finances the provision of care for medically complex children primarily through private health insurance coverage under employee-based group policy or an individual family policy. Recent studies, however, indicate that children make up a disproportionate share of the uninsured even as dependents of the employed (Blendon, 1982). In 1986, approximately 62% of American children between the ages of birth and 12, and only 50% of the technology-dependent children were covered by private insurance (Office of Technology Assessment, 1987). Moreover, this rate of coverage is correlated with family income such as that of the families with income below 200% of the federal poverty level, only 14% of the children are covered by private insurance (Office of Technology Assessment, 1987).

Of the families whose children are included in their insurance plan, a large proportion are not protected against the costs of a catastrophic illness, such as those incurred with the birth and long-term care of a medically complex child. Approximately 45% of American families are not adequately covered for such an event. Most long-term chronic disease care, home care and other services for children are excluded

Table 17.1. Private and Public Programs which Finance Services for Medically Complex Children.

Program	Eligibility	Coverage	State Participation
PRIVATE			
Third-party insurance	Employment or income to purchase individual policy	Varies by state regulations and policy	All states
Charitable organizations	Varies by organization	Varies according to condition or population	Depends on organizational scope or outreach
PUBLIC			
Maternal and child health block grant			
Children with special health needs (CSHN)	Determined by state, usually disability and income requirements	Variable, most states perform screening and treatment, case management and support for special needs children	All states
SPRANS demonstration grants	By application to MCHB/USPHS/DHHS	Varies by grant	Available to all
Medicaid	Based on income; mandatory coverage for AFDC and SSI recipients, pregnant women and children <100% of poverty	Financial coverage for medical care	All—federal match varies from 50%–80%, based on state per capita income

Program	Eligibility	Services	Coverage
Early and periodic screening diagnosis treatment (EPSDT)—mandatory	Medicaid eligible children <21	On-going screening, diagnosis and treatment	All states
Medically needy—optional	Not >133% of AFDC—determined by State	Same as basic Medicaid program	38 states
Foster/Adoptive Children—Optional	All state-placed, non-AFDC eligible	Same as basic Medicaid program	All states
Pregnant women and children—optional	All <185% poverty	Same as basic Medicaid program	All states
Home and community based waivers (HCB)	Medicaid eligible who would require long-term hospital care; plus expands eligibility limits	Homemaker, respite, home modifications, transportation, etc.	47 states
Model waivers	Same as HCB waivers, max 200 clients per waiver	Determined by state	26 states
TEFRA	SSI eligible children <21	All Medicaid services	32 states
COBRA (1985)	Medicaid eligible	Case management	All states
Medicare and catastrophic Care Act of 1988	Medicaid eligible infants <1 in "disproportionate share" hospitals	Provides option to states to extend inpatient day limits	All states
Medicare	Children <18 with end stage renal disease	Maintenance dyalisis, transplant surgery, physicians services	All states
CHAMPUS	Military personnel and family	Medical, drugs and limited home health, nursing care, and equipment	All states

from coverage (Blendon, 1982). In general, there is a poor match between the coverage from most insurance plans and the patterns of cost generated by a chronic illness (Hobbs, Perrin, & Ireys, 1985): Moreover, where there is coverage, it is typically only for hospital or other sophisticated technological care, and not for less costly alternatives such as home care, thereby encouraging more expensive, short-term patterns of care (Hobbs, Perrin, & Ireys, 1985) that requires substantial out-of-pocket payment by the family (Task Force, 1988).

The extent of coverage and amount required out-of-pocket varies according to insurer and insurance plan. For the medically-complex child, the most important features of a private health insurance plan are plan maximums (limits on the total paid by insurer), catastrophic stop-loss provisions (the upper limit on what the insured must pay out-of-pocket), and covered services (the limits on the amount, type and duration of services covered (Task Force, 1988). Recent trends indicate increases in overall plan maximums from $250,000 to $1 million or more, but an estimated 50% of all policies have inadequate coverage for the high cost of long-term care for technology-dependent children (Task Force, 1988). In terms of catastrophic stop-loss coverage, many plans have annual limits on a family's out-of-pocket expenses, but these plans do not prevent families from reaching their policy's lifetime maximum benefit limit and having their coverage withdrawn. Finally, few insurers cover the costs of home, nursing or respite care, important services for chronically ill children. Other, less obvious family issues are of concern as well. A family with a child who has special needs becomes a "wage slave" to the employer who holds the policy covering that family, i.e., if the employee wishes to change employers the issue of pre-existing illness becomes a significant factor in that the child's care will not be covered by a new employer. This fact constrains job choice in those families.

Recent initiatives for the care of the chronically ill have emerged from the private sector, including individual benefits management programs and waived maximum limits programs. In the first case, many services that were previously uncovered such as home services are paid for under the benefits management program if this coverage is expected to reduce overall benefit payments. In the second case, maximum spending limits are waived on a case-by-case basis. In addition, a few private insurers have considered increasing coverage for certain home care needs of the technology-dependent, such as for ventilator support or intravenous feeding technology. These expansions are rare and are not expected to become broadly available without legislative mandates.

If one views private insurance premiums as a "tax" for universally required service, then insurance premiums may be seen as an onerously regressive tax. Most employers offering health insurance set identical premium levels for all employees. Given a typical $4,000 per year premium for family coverage, an employee compensated $20,000 pays 20% of compensation on health insurance, while an employee compensated at $65,000 pays only 6% of compensation. This circumstance gives insight into the observation that coverage varies directly with income.

Charitable Organizations

It is estimated that more than twenty national charitable organizations, such as the March of Dimes and the National Easter Seals Society, provide research, services and funds for disabled children. The percentage of total outlays that each organization gives for direct services or family support varies from group to group ranging from 11% to 93%, and is dependent on the disability or handicap that is the concern of the organization (Task Force, 1988). For some medical problems, for instance, families may be provided funds for equipment or physical therapy, while children with other disabilities may not have access to such resources. For these reasons, charitable organizations are not viewed as a comprehensive or dependable source of financing for the care required of medically complex children. Moreover, the future role of such funding in the overall financing of care is viewed as declining as expansions in private and public health insurance, particularly for home care, ensue (Office of Technology Assessment, 1987). In general, funding through these agencies, though valuable, does not play a large role in the needed coordination of services and financing for the medically complex.

In summary, private third-party insurance represents an undeveloped funding resource for the care of medically complex children. With the development of expanded benefit packages and less stringent eligibility requirements, large group policies may offer the ability to spread the costs and risk of care for the chronically ill to a larger, more diverse group of people. But many changes are required before the private insurance option becomes viable for the medically complex. Some of the improvements needed include rates that are reasonably related to the actual costs of delivering benefits, promotion of the availability of full-benefit insurance at discounted rates for low-income families (a less regressive "tax"); waiting periods of no longer than six months for pre-existing conditions; the inclusion of case management services at no extra charge; and the option of "structured settlements in the form of medical trusts for the care of technology-dependent children" (Task Force, 1988). These steps, while still incremental approaches to improving access to care, would make appropriate care for the medically complex more available and would begin to mold private insurance coverage to the needs of chronically ill children and their families.

Public Sector Funding Sources

There is currently no comprehensive public system of care delivery or financing for handicapped children and their families in the U.S. Instead there are a number of separate programs and funding streams which are individually administered under separate federal legislation and appropriations. These programs include: 1) the Children with Special Health Care Needs (CSHN) program, previously called Crippled Children's Services; 2) Medicaid, including EPSDT; 3) Developmental Disabilities program; 4) Education of All Handicapped Children (P.L. 94-142 and P.L. 99-457) services; 5) CHAMPUS; and 6) special federal or state-financed programs, such as SSI, foster care, and Title XX. In addition, many charitable organizations provide services and funding for services for medically complex children. These programs are described below.

(1) Title V: Services for Children with Special Health Needs (CSHN)—
   In 1935, Title V, part 2 of the Social Security Act established the federal authorization for state Crippled Children's Programs, now called the program for Children with Special Health Needs (CSHN). This program was established to encourage a partnership between federal and state governments in the identification, evaluation, diagnosis, rehabilitation, and case management of handicapped children, youth and their families. Until the mid-1960's when Medicaid was established, the CSHN was the only source of public funding for low-income, chronically-ill children. In 1981, the Omnibus Budget Reconciliation Act established the Maternal and Child Health Block Grant which consolidated ten programs, including the CSHN, thereby allowing states greater discretion over

programs. Federal funds are allocated to state CSHN programs through a grant of $70,000, plus an additional amount matched by formula including both the number of children under 21 years of age and the financial ability of the state.

Currently, the Title V CSHN is the only program that provides for both the organization and financing of care. Moreover, many CSHN programs are required to work in coordination with the state's Medicaid program. Virtually any needed service may be covered by the CSHN, including case management, home care, nursing and respite care services, and coordination of services for children covered by Medicaid waivers. As such, it is one of the most important, albeit under-financed, programs for chronically ill children and their families (Task Force, 1988).

The Title V Special Projects of Regional and National Significance (SPRANS) grant program is also viewed as important to the development and financing of care for chronically ill children. In particular, some demonstration projects provide funding for the chronic care of children. Other projects have provided for systems of comprehensive, coordinated care. However, SPRANS grants are time limited and are typically used for demonstration.

Each state establishes program specifications for CSHN and, as a consequence, the program varies substantially among states. Typical limitations associated with the CSHN program, include nominal financing, stringent medical or financial eligibility criteria, limited service availability, and limited coordination with other programs. Potential means of alleviating these weaknesses that have been discussed include national, uniform expansion of program eligibility and outreach (both of which would provide greater access to this source of funding for the medically complex) and better planning and coordination with the Medicaid, Special Education and Developmental Disabilities Programs.

(2) Title XIX: Medicaid—Initially established in 1965 as Title XIX of the Social Security Act, Medicaid provides federal assistance to states to pay for medical services for financially and medically needy persons. Federal Medicaid dollars are provided as a match to state dollars, with the match varying from 50% to 80% depending on the state's per capita income. Medicaid consists of numerous mandatory and optional coverage categories resulting in a complex web of eligibility and related programs that vary from state to state. The eligibility groups that all states must cover are: Aid to Families with Dependent Children (AFDC) recipients,

certain blind and disabled persons, certain poverty-related pregnant women and children, and Supplemental Security Income (SSI) recipients. Optional programs include: children receiving state supplements, medically needy, foster and adoptive children, non-poverty pregnant women and children, and special waiver recipients. All of these programs are critical to the financing of care for very low-income medically complex children and their families as they provide financial and medical aid that would otherwise not be received.

Services that all states are required to provide are hospitalization, laboratory services, rural health clinic services, physician services, and Early and Periodic Screening Diagnosis and Treatment (EPSDT) for children, but states may also offer up to 32 additional services, including home care or nursing care, home respiratory care, and case management. States are given considerable flexibility in the Medicaid programs, e.g., they determine eligibility thresholds, payment rates and standards for providers and services. These state-level programmatic options, however, have created a complex, piecemeal, system for low-income children needing Medicaid services (Hobbs et al., 1985). Moreover, most state Medicaid program do not provide the range of services required by medically complex children because of the costs or administrative difficulties of adding these provisions to their program. For example, the Medicaid 2176 Home and Community-Based Waivers, available to states for the funding of a variety of home and community support services, is one program that is capable of bringing relief to many low-income families of chronically ill children. Such waivers are not universally available because of the cost and lengthy process of application and renewal. When available, these waivers may provide Medicaid recipients and their families with funding for services including home modifications, habilitation and respite care. Currently, most of these waivers are used for elderly or mentally-retarded people and rarely for medically complex children. The development and use of such waivers as they apply to medically complex children would be a significant step for many states.

Similar to statewide waivers, "Model" Home and Community Based Waivers are designed to encourage state to provide funding for services to targeted groups of chronically ill children and adults. Most important for the chronically ill, these waivers allow states to waive SSI financial eligibility rules to permit Medicaid eligibility for non-institutional services. Their main drawback is that states are limited within each waiver to offering services to no more than 200 persons per year. However, there is no apparent limit on the number of such waivers which may be obtained. It should be noted that both the Home and Community-Based Waivers and the Model Waivers programs were fashioned after the earlier, so-called "Katie Beckett" Waiver program. The latter was a make-shift program designed to accommodate the needs of one child per application. That program, no longer available, was established by Presidential fiat during the first term of the Reagan administration in response to unstinting administrative and political efforts on the part of the parents of an Iowa preschooler, after whom the waiver was named.

Two provisions under Medicaid are worthy of special note: (1) an amendment under TEFRA of 1982 which allows states to provide regular Medicaid coverage, without a waiver, to certain categories of disabled children living at home; (2) the Medicaid Early Periodic Screening, Diagnosis and Treatment (EPSDT) program. The EPSDT program was a 1968 amendment to Title XIX of the Social Security Act which requires states to: (1) identify and diagnose health problems in children; (2) to make arrangements for treatments for children in need; and (3) to encourage regular participation in the health care system.

In recent years Congress has added coverage for a number of benefits and groups under Medicaid that have been important for medically complex children. These include: P.L. 99-272 in 1985 which allows states to offer case management services to targeted populations; P.L. 99-509 which permits states to cover at-home respiratory care services to ventilator dependent children and adults without obtaining a waiver; P.L. 100-203 which optionally extends eligibility for children up to age 6 in states; and through OBRA's 1987's extension of optional Medicaid eligibility to pregnant women and their families with income up to 185% of poverty. All of these recent amendments have provided additional avenues for states to reach the medically complex children through Medicaid. Because states have the option to not adopt these improvements children in many states are left without coverage that could be obtained in neighboring states, and the coverage available remains too limited to compensate for many of the services required by the families of children who are medically complex.

(3) Developmental Disabilities—The Developmental Disabilities Act
(P.L. 100-146) assists states in developing comprehensive and coordinated services for persons with developmental disabilities. All
persons who became dependent on technological devices before
age 22 qualify as developmentally disabled under this act, and are
able to access the programs offered. Through these programs, this
Act provides funding to states to provide a system of individualized services and stimulate the development of interdisciplinary
training and research on developmental disabilities, and to protect
the legal and human rights of developmentally disabled persons.
These programs are beneficial in the provision of funding for
services for the developmentally disabled and in the protection
of their rights, but are limited in the amount of medical care
services they cover.

(4) Education of All Handicapped Children (P.L. 94-142 & P.L. 99-
457)—The Education for all Handicapped Children Act of 1975
(Public Law 94-142), implemented nationally in 1977, requires
public schools to implement procedures aimed at the identification, evaluation, classroom placement, and individualized curric-
ular planning for students with physical, learning or emotional
disabilities (Palfrey, Singer, Walker & Butler, 1986). This act
places responsibility for instruction and any "related services" for
every handicapped child in the hands of the public schools, and
calls for the identification of federal, state, local and private resources available within states to support these services (Fox,
Freedman & Klepper, 1988).

Building on P.L. 94-142 which provided for the provision of a
free, appropriate, public education for all handicapped children,
P.L. 99-457 expanded the federal assistance to states to plan for
a system of educational and related services for handicapped pre-
school children, including funding for early intervention services
for children ages birth to three, and special education and related
services to children three to five. These laws are significant for
medically complex children not only because of the funding and
public oversight committed by the government to these issues,
but also because of the broad range of services that are financed.
These include family training, counseling, speech and hearing
therapy, occupational and physical therapy, case management,
and "health services necessary to enable the child to benefit from
other early intervention services" (Fox, Freedman & Klepper,
1988). The success of states in providing such comprehensive

services to handicapped children, however, lies in their ability to access both public and private financial resources. Recommended actions to secure such financial support include the legislative expansion of public funding and private insurance policies to cover the services outlined in P.L. 99-457 (Fox, Freedman, & Klepper, 1988).

(5) CHAMPUS—The Department of Defense provides health care for family members of military personnel through the Civilian Health and Medical Program of the Uniformed Services (CHAMPUS) by sharing in the costs of care not available to these families through military treatment facilities. CHAMPUS financing of care for medically complex children is available through either "regular home health benefits," which include coverage of medical equipment oxygen, parenteral and enteral nutrition therapies, skilled nursing care and medications, or through the "Program for the Handicapped," which provides financial assistance when a member's mentally retarded or seriously physically handicapped dependents are excluded from public programs. Benefits of this latter program include diagnostic services, inpatient, outpatient, rehabilitation, special education, durable medical equipment, supplies and skilled nursing, but the benefits are limited to $1,000 per month and all services must be approved in advance. Neither program is designed to adequately address the needs of medically complex children.

Though coverage through these programs is adequate for initial equipment and service needs of medically complex children, in the long-term these resources are largely inadequate for this population because of the monthly spending maximums and limited community services. Moreover, CHAMPUS regulations prohibit the coverage of "custodial care" (defined as care rendered to a patient who has a physical or mental disability that is expected to be prolonged, requires a monitored environment, either at home or in an institution), or who requires assistance to support the essentials of daily living (Task Force, 1988). This limitation effectively prohibits the coverage of care for many medically complex and most technology-dependent children. Military families with medically complex children, therefore, face a challenge in the acquisition of long-term care.

(6) Special Services—Special services or cash benefit programs that medically complex children and their families may qualify for include Supplemental Security Income (SSI), the adoption and

foster care incentive program, and in-home services under Title XX Social Services Block Grants. Each of these programs is tied to income and disability eligibility. For example, cash benefits and state supplementary payments are available to non-institutionalized disabled individuals whose low income qualifies them for SSI benefits; and in-home services, including a home health aide or transportation, are available to low-income individuals. While these state-based programs are "gap-filling" for many children and families in need, these variable, categorical programs are limited in their ability to provide comprehensive, long-term services or financing. Moreover, the quality, interagency coordination, and universal accessibility of such funding is limited because these programs are state-specific (Task Force, 1988).

Overall, the Task Force (1987) noted a number of specific barriers in the provision of public services and financing for medically complex children. These include: (1) lack of national policy commitment to needs of children; (2) federal and state government reluctance to replace charitable care; (3) insecurity of continued public and private financing sources making future planning problematic for states; (4) unavailability of accessible information on state financed and waiver programs; and (5) complex rules for federal Medicaid waivers making this option difficult to understand and implement.

Public and Private Cooperatives

The major cooperative arrangements among private and public organizations in the provision of funding to the chronically ill are state health insurance risk pools. These pools, currently operating in seven states but legislatively approved in fifteen, are organizations of private insurers coordinated by the state to serve the needs of a special population of medically needy, formerly known as "uninsurables." To be eligible for coverage through state pools, persons must have been rejected by one or two private insurers for coverage, face premiums that exceed those of the high risk pool, have received a notice of benefit reduction because of pre-existing condition, or have a certain chronic condition (Griss, 1989). These pools provide a valuable service not available to many chronically ill. The concentration of high-risk participants into a common pool, however, presents a financial challenge to states that have organized such pools because the costs to the state and to individuals still run high. For example, individual premiums run about 150%–400% of standard premiums, deductibles range from $1000 to $2000, and enrollee co-payments can be 20% of all covered services (Griss, 1989). Moreover, contrary to the legislation that established them, most pools do not provide more comprehensive coverage or greater arrays of services than standard policies. For example, high risk pools do not often pay for home health care, durable medical equipment, or physical therapy on an on-going basis; moreover, many of them have lifetime maximum benefits of $250,000 (Griss, 1989). With the deficits mounting among state high-risk pools, and the reality of the inability of these pools to reach many of the "hard core" uninsurables, restructuring is required before these pools can adequately meet the needs of the medically complex population. Specifically, the broadening of the risk pools and the improved management of the enrollee's medical spending are potential avenues for improving the viability of these pools in providing coverage for the chronically ill.

ALTERNATIVE FINANCING STRATEGIES

A number of alternative strategies for funding the care of medically complex children have been recommended or implemented in recent years. These are outlined below.

Private Sector Alternatives

While numerous expansions in individual insurance policies have been discussed in recent years to make private insurance coverage more responsive to the needs of the medically complex, few alternative programs have emerged. One concept that has been discussed is that of medical trusts which would provide funding for the chronically ill through the interest earned or invested trusts. In these the insurer would anticipate the lifelong cost of care and provide a principal amount in trust, which would generate sufficient interest to cover the annual cost of care. With the initial investment of a large sum, private insurers could guarantee coverage of benefits paid through the interest earned while the principal amount would be maintained.

Public Sector Alternatives

The largest number of recently proposed strategies for the funding of care for the medically complex have been in the public sector. Examples of these, as noted earlier, include Medicaid waivers and state-financed catastrophic coverage programs. Though fragmented and limited in coverage, these programs provide a foundation for the development of additional financing. A publicly financed strategy recently proposed to expand the funding and delivery of appropriate services is the utilization of the Medicaid program to assume responsibility for coordinating care for medically complex children. Through Medicaid's EPSDT service authority, Medicaid agencies would negotiate an individualized prepaid fee to cover services, administration, and stop-loss insurance through a state-certified organization for the delivery of appropriate care for children. Collections from other liable third party-payers and families would also be sought, but Medicaid would remain "administratively responsible for providing access to systematically coordinated care for all technology-dependent children, without regard to their financial eligibility" (Task Force, 1988).

The choice of Medicaid to administer such a program was intended to assure a government role in quality control and to avoid new federal legislation. Legislation would be required, however, to waive Medicaid eligibility and freedom-of-choice provisions to permit states to negotiate a prepaid fee per child with qualified organizations. Additionally, private insurance and family financial participation in costs for care would have to be legislatively authorized. This plan was favored by the Task Force because it utilized existing public and private structures, assured greater access to all in need regardless of financial ability, and assured some degree of quality control.

Public and Private Cooperative Alternatives

The development of national programs to provide comprehensive services or financing to medically complex children through the coordination of private and public efforts seems to hold the greatest hope of policy makers and health policy analysts (Blendon, 1982, Hobb et al., 1985; Task Force, 1988). A number of such programs have recently been proposed. For instance, in June the U.S. Senate Finance Committee proposed the funding of demonstration projects to study the effect on access to health care, private insurance coverage, and costs of health care when states are allowed to extend benefits under Medicaid to children who, because of a pre-existing medical condition or the exhaustion of private health insurance benefits, can be considered to be medically uninsurable (Congressional Record, S 6892). These projects would extend Medicaid eligibility to families with chronically ill children who a) are less than 6 years old with a family income less than 185% of poverty; or b) are between 6 and 20 and in a family with income less than 100% of poverty, through the collection of premiums from families with incomes between 100% and 200% of poverty. Families with less than 100% of poverty would not be required to pay premiums, while those between 100% and 200% of poverty would pay either the actuarial value of the coverage or 3 percent of the families monthly earnings; and those with income over 200% of poverty would pay a premium equal to the actuarial value of the coverage. In addition, one of the proposed demonstration projects will evaluate the feasibility of employer contributions to the premiums. Such demonstrations should provide important information concerning the costs of such expansions, the changes in access to care for these populations, and the effects of employer and beneficiary Medicaid buy-in on Medicaid utilization and costs.

Another national plan, which would utilize the public and private sector in the development of alternative health insurance policies and funding, was recently outlined by Freedman, et al. (1988). To enhance access to health care for children and their family members, school systems would be used as grouping mechanisms for negotiating comprehensive group health insurance policies. Coverage would be offered to all families with children enrolled in public school. Policies could be designed to accommodate either the individual child or the entire family. Premiums would be on a sliding scale based on ability to pay. Such flexibility would be ideally suited to the needs of parents who receive individual coverage as a fringe benefit of employment, but who must pay a relatively large premium for supplemental family coverage. This arrangement is identical to current employment-based insurance structures, except that school children become the "employees," qualifying both themselves and their family members for coverage. A health insurance program based on school enrollment could be structured to target three groups: the uninsured, the under-insured, and those for whom the program would represent an economically competitive choice. Though the benefit package would be the same for all participants, the enticement for each group might be different.

If reasonably priced, this comprehensive health insurance program would afford access to coverage for the uninsured, better coverage for the under-insured, and a better buy for the economically secure. Indeed, for families in which the wage earner already receives employment-based coverage, the option of coverage for the child only through school-based insurance might be a low cost alternative to the purchase of employment-based coverage for the family. The size of the risk pool generated by such a plan would be capable of accommodating the extraordinary costs associated with medically complex children without jeopardizing the actuarial soundness of the risk pool. This demonstration, as well as the others, through their utilization of public and private agencies are designed to be models for future statewide health insurance plans for all children.

The development of additional public-private financing cooperatives to provide better coverage of care for families of chronically ill children, as well as all children, are urgently needed. As with the above programs, alternatives that utilize the resources (i.e., funding and care systems) of both public and private organizations offer the greatest potential of keeping costs low and of providing comprehensive and coordinated care rather than individual piecemeal programs available today.

CONCLUSION

A review of the mechanisms of financing care for medically complex children unfolds numerous and interrelated challenges to the provision of appropriate, accessible medical care for medically complex children. Most significantly, there is no existing system that provides adequately for the needs of these children and their families. In addition, where coverage is available, information about accessing the services is often not provided. This is particularly true for respite care, home health care, and case management services. Moreover, the many gaps found in the delivery of care to chronically ill children indicates significant deficits in the provision of funding currently available through the public and private sectors. For example, even Medicaid waivers and eligibility expansions have failed to adequately meet the needs of medically complex children and their families.

It is clear, therefore, that piecemeal health care financing solutions for small segments of our population are and will remain unable to adequately serve the growing population of medically complex children and their families. The cause of this inability, as we have presented above, lies not only in the inadequacies of current systems of care financing but also in the lack of both comprehensive and coordinated care through existing programs. Because access to health care is inextricably tied to financing systems, the improvement of both access and adequacy of services to medically complex children will depend on the development of coordinated systems of care that utilize current care providers and new sources of financing and delivery. Moreover, to keep these systems affordable, efficient mechanisms for coordinating care and accessing funding, such as through large pools of payors, must be in place. The means of achieving such goals, therefore, are found in increased attention to the needs of the medically complex population and in the coordination of public and private efforts in order to avoid duplicative and/or inadequate services. Recurrent calls for universal access to health care and the efforts of health care professionals in the call for improved and coordinated systems of care through policy and program changes are hopeful signs that the needs of special health populations will be met. Failing universal access, children with special needs and their families will continue to be petitioners for extraordinary consideration and will continue to be disappointed.

REFERENCES

Blendon, R. J. (1982). Paying for medical care for children: A continuing financial dilemma. In *Financing Pediatric Care*. Year Book Medical Publishers, Inc.

Butler, J. A., Winter, W. D., Singer, J. D., & Wenger, M. (1985). Medical care use and expenditure among children and youth in the United States: Analysis of a national probability sample. *Pediatrics, 76*, 495–507.

Fox, H. B., Freedman, S. A., & Klepper, B. R. (1989). Financing programs for young children with handicaps. In J. J. Gallagher, P. L. Trohanis, & R. M. Clifford (Eds.), *Policy Implementation & P.L. 99-457: Planning for young children with special needs* (pp. 169–182). Baltimore, MD: Paul H. Brooks Publishing.

Freedman, S. A., Klepper, B. R., Duncan, R. P., & Bell, S. P. (1988). Coverage of the uninsured and underinsured: A proposal for school enrollment-based family health insurance. *The New England Journal of Medicine, 318*(13), 843–847.

General Accounting Office. (1989). *Health care: Home care experiences of families with chronically ill children.* (GAO/HRD-89-73). Washington, DC: Author.

Griss, B. (1989). *Access to health care.* (Policy Bulletin—12/88–3/89). Washington, DC: World Institute on Disability.

Hobbs, N., Perrin, J. M., & Ireys, H. T. (1985). *Chronically ill children and their families.* San Francisco: Jossey-Bass Publishers.

Newacheck, P. W., Budetti, P. P., & McManus, P. (1984). Trends in childhood disability. *American Journal of Public Health, 74*(3), 232–236.

Office of Technology Assessment, U.S. Congress. (1987). *Technology-Dependent Children: Hospital v. Home Care—A Technical Memorandum* (Office of Technology Assessment-TM-H-38). Washington, DC: U.S. Government Printing Office.

Select Panel for the Promotion of Child Health. (1981). *Better health for children: A national strategy.* (DHHS Publication No. 79-55071.) Washington, DC: U.S. Government Printing Office.

Task Force on Technology-Dependent Children (1988). *Fostering Home and Community-Based Care for Technology-Dependent Children.* Department of Health and Human Services.

Walker, D. K., Palfrey, J. S., Butler, J. A., & Singer, J. (1988). Use and source of payment for health and community services for children with impaired mobility. *Public Health Reports, 103*(4), 411–415.

Section VIII
Outcomes

CHAPTER 18

STRESS AND COPING IN HOME CARE: A STUDY OF FAMILIES*

KATHLEEN E. MURPHY

INTRODUCTION

The father of a quadriplegic, ventilator assisted child spoke quietly:

> Over the last year especially—I get depressed at how this has gotten to us . . . we've lost years of our lives to this . . . vacations, building a home, having good times as a family—those days are gone for good and there isn't a way out . . . finally it has hit me that this is permanent and we'll end up with a 40 year old in our house who is handicapped and that has been our whole life.

An older sister summed up the realities of her life at home with a sister who is ventilator dependent:

> Everyone spends so much time with her that I have to be perfect so things run smooth. No one wants to have to pay attention to me. . . . I don't ask much and I get the small end of the bargain anyway. She gets everything first and I'm last on the list. I think it's to prove to her that they still love her—I guess I think it's because I'm older and because I'm not handicapped.

These comments by family members of children who are ventilator assisted are not isolated feelings. These are children who have survived because of advancements in medical technology—technology which has achieved the ability to provide *quantity* of life for the child without addressing the question of the *quality* of life for the family. It was the intent of this study to explore the perceptions of family members of such children living at home. The specific focus was on identifying those factors which were perceived as causing stress, what the effects of the stress were on family functioning, and how family

*This work was funded in part by MCH-DHHS SPRANS Grant No 5173363.

members coped with the stress. Because the focus was "stress," these data do present a somewhat more pessimistic view of home care than may be found in some of the clinical accounts of the discharge planning process which emphasize the virtue of home over hospital (Goldberg, 1984). The following is not intended to dissuade families or the health care system from care at home. It is intended to portray the practical reality of what families will face in order to better prepare them.

LITERATURE REVIEW

In the present study, stress theory from a family systems perspective was used as a basis for looking at the experience of pediatric home ventilation. Within this paradigm, stress refers to any agent or force that threatens the well-being of any member of the family, thereby threatening the dynamic equilibrium of the entire system (Shonkoff, Jarman, & Kohlenberg, 1987). As such, the stress as that found in having a ventilated child, would affect every member of the family (McCubbin & Patterson, 1983; Brown, 1984). However, empirical studies of stress for families of children who are ventilator assisted are, to date, non-existent. Nonetheless, a number of studies of the families of children with other chronic conditions such as cerebral palsy (Coffman, 1983), diabetes (Hodges & Parker, 1987), cancer (Barbarin, Hughes, & Chesler, 1985), renal failure (Reynolds, 1986), cystic fibrosis (McCubbin, 1984) and mental retardation (Blacher, 1984; Frederick & Frederick, 1981) have found that the families experience: (1) social isolation; (2) financial burden; (3) disrupted marital and sibling relationships; (4) difficulties in activities of daily living due to caretaking responsibilities or medical appointments; (5) emotional reactions of grief, anger, disappointment, and guilt; and (6) a lack of information regarding community resources. The lack of co-ordination of clinic visits, physician appointments, and community resources add to the disruption of daily life and planning for the future (Lyon & Preis, 1983; Yoos, 1987). Emerging clinical accounts of home care for technology dependent children suggest additional stressors: the chronicity and unpredictability of medical crises; adjustment to in-home staff; and uneven services from home care providers such as nursing agencies and equipment vendors (Feinberg, 1986; Weinstock, 1986; OTA, 1987). The literature regarding the impact of other chronic conditions on the affected child include concerns about: (1) the body including image, function, and limitations; (2) the disabling condition, e.g., restrictions on lifestyles, information, and death; (3) the future; (4) social isolation; (5) prolonged dependency on parents and health care providers; and (6) emotional reactions including feelings of inadequacy, anxiety, depression, and embarrassment. (Coffman, 1983; Hamburg, 1974; Litt, Cuskey & Rosenberg, 1982; Travis, 1976). While there is little research in the area of sibling adjustment to having a handicapped brother or sister at home, of the clinical articles which address the siblings' experience the focus is almost exclusively on the relationship of siblings to parents (McKeever, 1983) and emphasizes the negative effects of decreased parental time and attention (Featherstone, 1980; McHale, Simeonsson & Sloan, 1984; Teiber, Mabe & Wilson, 1987). Other studies have found both positive and negative effects including: increased tolerance for differences in others; higher levels of empathy and altruism; increased sense of maturity; guilt for being healthy; fear of catching the chronic condition; feelings of being neglected by parents; school maladjustment; and resentment of attention given to the handicapped sibling. Sibling stress may also be surmised from reports of somatic problems, including sleep disturbances, enuresis, eating disorders, headaches, recurrent abdominal pain, and preoccupation with health (McKeever, 1983; Powell & Ogle, 1985).

Within the family literature, McCubbin and Patterson (1983) identified five factors which mediate how a family copes with stress, including: acquiring social support from relatives and friends; reframing and redefining stressful events to make them manageable; spiritual support; acquiring help from the community; and passive appraisal of problematic issues to minimize reactivity. Numerous authors affirm the importance of social support from within the circle of family and friends as well as the community (Turner, 1983; McCubbin, M., 1984; Stuifbergen, 1987). These authors also cite certain personality characteristics and general attitudes as mediators of stress and an influence on the use of various coping efforts. A number of studies identify specific coping strategies used by families of chronically ill children which tend to be similar to those identified by McCubbin et al. with one addition: "information seeking" as a frequently used coping strategy (Coffman, 1983; Barbarin et al., 1985; Horner, Rawlins & Giles, 1987).

METHODOLOGY AND SAMPLE

In order to develop a comprehensive model of discharge and home care planning for ventilator assisted children, an exploratory research study was designed to interview the "experts"—the families caring for their children at home. Seventy-four percent of the available sample of families (n = 21 families and n = 28 parent interviews) participated in the study. With the exception of race, (the sample was 95% caucasian) the demographics of the sample of parent respondents mirrored a normal population of families in Illinois in age, income, education, employment and so on.

FINDINGS

Stressors in Home Care

> I have had times where I wanted to sleep until it was all over . . . I just wanted to go to bed and have everything taken care of . . . every once in a while—Oh, when I get real exhausted from taking care of him a lot without a nurse—I think I'll just go to sleep and forget about this for a while. . . .

Parents were asked to think back on the early months of being at home and to identify those areas of home care for which the discharge planning process may not have prepared them. Twenty-five parents indicated that the most difficult aspect of home care was dealing with the home care nursing. At the time of the study, 19 families had nurses from five to seven days a week and from 12 to 24 hours a day. Forty-eight percent of those families were receiving nursing services 24 hours a day, seven days a week. All those in homes with nurses had experienced problems and no parents identified fewer than three distinct problem areas. While seven parents (28%, representing six families) complained of poorly trained nurses or of poor nursing care, this problem was not primary. Most frequently mentioned were: nurses' disrespect for parental authority (64%); loss of privacy (48%); basic personality differences with parents and/or child (48%); inconsistency of staffing (36%); and general laziness or not doing the complete job (32%). Parents felt "judged" by nurses regarding: discipline of the other children (24%); relationships between family members, particularly spousal or dating relationships (24%); religious or spiritual values (12%); and alcohol use (12%). Other more minor complaints included nurses using the phone for long distance calls, opening family mail, going through personal papers and drawers, not cleaning up after themselves, or slamming the door when entering and leaving at shift change. All other stressors paled beside the complex issue of home care nurses as parents also freely admitted they could not "do" home care without the nurses. The following comment is indicative of the overall feeling of parents in having nurses in the home:

> They don't take it as a job because it's somebody's home. The disrespect we feel we have gotten from nurses has just been more to handle than my child's situation in its entirety.

A second source of stress was the financial situation created by home care. Ten parents (representing eight families, 40%) had private insurance, 17 parents (representing eleven families, 55%) had only public aid coverage and one parent (5%) had a combination of public aid and insurance to cover the cost of home care and medical expenses. It was originally believed that the funding differed between public and private sources and that the difference would result in fewer services for publicly funded families. This did not turn out to be true as all parents generally felt their private insurance or state public aid adequately covered the direct costs of the child's medical care. Further, parents did not feel that the quality of the care received by the child was markedly different under public aid compared to insurance but three felt that cutbacks in nursing hours required by public aid were going to affect the care in the future.

Some parents mentioned the indirect costs which were not covered by either public or private funding. These included increased utility bills, general wear and tear on the home and increased cost of paper items (paper towels, tissues, toilet paper, etc.) because of the additional people in the home. While the financial plan which enabled parents to take their ventilated child home was generally adequate in covering the medical care of the child, the out-of-pocket expenses decreased resources available to the family for other activities and required changes in employment status and lifestyle.

The final stressor had to do with the emotional/psychological components of home care. As the study progressed, however, it became clear that the "home care situation" and the "feelings" about the child and family were significantly intertwined and interdependent with other stresses. Therefore, findings about parents' feelings are presented with the speculation that parents' feelings about their situation are both a cause and a result of stress. Parents were asked about feelings found in the literature to be common in parents with children with a chronic illness. While the ventilated children are not "ill," ventilator assistance is a chronic handicapping condition and an assumption was made that some of the feeling content of home care might be similar.

All of the parents in this study acknowledged having difficult feelings about having a technology assisted child at home including: periodic depression (85%); anger (78%); and anxiety about the future (70%). Another difficult feeling for parents and an aspect of loss which is related to depression and sadness was "chronic sorrow." Eighteen parents (64%) spoke of a periodic, ongoing sense of loss of the child who used to be or who would have been if something had not intervened. For example:

> I do when I see young girls, like when we go to the bowling alley or going out to the fairs, and I see a young girl with long blonde hair. . . . I don't know how to explain it. . . . I don't wish this on that girl but I wish my daughter was that girl.

All parents who experienced this sort of loss said it was most likely to occur when around other children but not all the time. As one parent said: "when it does happen it is quite unexpected." Some parents said that birthdays were hard but birthdays, holidays, and anniversaries did not seem to serve as stimuli for these thoughts as consistently as the occasion of simply being around other children.

Sixteen parents (59%) also acknowledged having felt "guilt" related to the child's condition. Eleven (69%) felt that there was something they or their spouse did or did not do which could have protected the child from the condition. Parents whose child needed to be ventilated at birth were more likely to experience guilt but only for the time after the birth (less than one year). All but one of these mothers talked of guilt related to her actions during pregnancy but felt they had been able to get beyond feeling guilty. However, parents whose child had an accident talked of a more pervasive and ongoing sense of guilt lasting years. Parents also discussed experiencing other aspects of guilt which were different from the guilt of having caused the child's condition. For example:

> I feel guilty because I feel different about (older sibling) and (child)— I like (older sibling) better. (Child) was taken away from me at birth, that's the only way I can rationalize it. She was taken away from me and she wasn't my baby until she was six months old and then for only two weeks—and then she was my 'dying baby' and then she was my

healthy baby and then my dying baby . . . I don't feel as close to her—
I think it's unfair and I try not to make it show. . . .

Lastly, thirteen parents (48%) felt socially and emotionally isolated by the experience. For example:

Seems like there's hundreds of people going through the house but people don't invite us over because (child) can't come. This whole thing has really isolated us because he can't be up. We rely on family for our support.

It was thought that in addition to the other feelings, parents would have anxiety about the possibility of the child dying. While thoughts of the child dying were there for many parents (57%), they kept these thoughts on the "back burner" rather than focus on them. They seemed to achieve a certain level of acceptance of the possibility and then did not dwell on it.

The Effects of Stress on Family Relationships

Parents were asked what changes they had experienced in the marital relationship since the child came home. Twenty-two of the parents were married at the time of the study. Of the thirteen spouses (59%) who felt there had been changes for the better in the marital relationship, seven (54%) felt the husband and wife were "closer." For example:

We are much closer now, we tend to take life more seriously. Big problems or little problems don't seem to matter as much. If everyone is happy and if he is fine nothing else matters. Our priorities have changed.

Of the thirteen spouses (59%) who felt there were changes for the worse, a number mentioned problems with distance or lack of support. For example:

The care of (child) feels like it's more important than I am. The result is a protective wall kind—so there are times of getting close which you know can only go so far—you'll be too emotionally involved and angry when the reality that she (wife) will have to go and take care of (child) comes back.

When asked what the most difficult adjustment had been for the couple, ten spouses (77%) mentioned the loss of privacy due to nurses which made it difficult to talk, argue or be sexual. Other adjustments mentioned included: how to discipline the ventilated child without being overly protective; dealing with having a handicapped child; loss of freedom; and having less time to spend with other family members. Nonetheless, when asked to compare the quality of the marriage "now" with the marriage "before" (the child's condition began), 73% of spouses felt the marriage was the same or better. It is also significant to note that there were no couples which had divorced since home care began.

Parents were also asked about changes they may have undergone as parents. The seven parents for whom the ventilated child was the first or only child, were unsure whether they would be different had the child not been ventilated. Of the remaining 21 parents, sixteen (76%) felt that they do things differently as parents. An overriding theme related to, in one parent's words, "becoming more 'go with the flow.' " For example:

> I'm a lot nicer. I try to make quality time better because I don't have much quantity. I try to do more things with the kids, let the house go or eat later in order to do things with the kids—I'm not so rigid about the house as I used to be.

> You learn what is 'emergency' and what is not an emergency—I don't react as much anymore—I'm much more tolerant and patient than I used to be—If it's not life threatening then there's no reason to get bent out of shape.

Thirteen of the 21 parents (62%) with other children felt their relationship with the other children had been changed by home care. For some the change was in not having enough time for the others while other parents felt the relationship was closer because the siblings were more accessible than the ventilated child. It is interesting to note that only fathers felt they had a closer relationship with the other children. Mothers were more likely to express frustration and regret at the distance imposed by having to spend so much time and attention on the ventilated child at the expense of the other children.

Parents were asked to consider the effect the siblings ("normal" and ventilated) seemed to have on each other. Eighteen out of 21 (86%) parents who had other children felt the ventilated child had a positive effect on the other siblings in terms of their having to learn patience and to mature more quickly. In addition, twenty parents (95%) were able to identify positive effects of the other children on the ventilated child in regard to providing more "normal" relationships. Sixteen parents (76%) identified some negative effects of the ventilated child on siblings. However, none of the comments made regarding negative effects were directly related to the child but rather to the care of the child in the home, e.g., impact of nurses, the attention the child requires, etc. For example:

> They get put on the shelf an awful lot. Like now, Mike is going into the seventh grade and we were supposed go to the school for orientation. It's on the day Mary goes in for surgery. Ordinary families have this to some degree; we have it all the time. She is always first. And if you are in a play and something happens, that's tough. Everybody's tired of that. Many nurses and agencies are not sympathetic to that at all. I understand Mary's situation is more important, but it's always more important and it's not fair.

According to the parents', all family relationships: marital, parent-child, and sibling were changed by the experience of pediatric home care but definitely not all negatively. While these data must be interpreted cautiously, the parents' perceptions were certainly more positive than anticipated.

The Effects of Stress on Family Activities

The researcher had expected social isolation and loss of freedom due to the demands of home care to result in a decrease in the activities in which individuals and families would be able to engage. Twenty parents (71%) felt home care had caused them to decrease their level of activity. The primary reason given was that "you can't just pick up and go somewhere. It takes a lot of planning and thought to do anything. There can be no spontaneity." Included in the concept of 'thought and planning' were efforts which had to be made by parents in order to leave home. If the child was going to go along, access for wheelchairs had to be determined, available electrical and emergency services in the event of a mechanical breakdown had to be identified, the trip had to be scheduled around nursing shift changes, and it was a hassle just having to take along all of the necessary equipment. If the child was not going to go along, the parent had to make arrangements for the care of the other children, make sure they could be reached at all times in the event of an emergency, and that there was adequate staff coverage for the child. Other reasons given for the decreases in activity included no money and less time for as many activities but these considerations were minor compared to the planning and preparation aspect. Several parents stated they did more together earlier in home care but it had gotten to be too much work and the activity level had decreased over time.

Coping with Stress and the Effects of Stress

At the beginning of the study it was thought that if the specific strategies used by "veteran" parents to cope with home care could be identified, similar strategies could be taught to "new" parents just entering home care. Throughout each section of the interview dealing with stress, family members were asked how they specifically dealt with stress. They were also asked a series of questions about what internal qualities or life experiences they felt might have helped them to cope.

Twenty-two (78%) parents felt a number of life experiences or combinations of life experiences had been helpful, including: the death of a family member; having a disabled member in the family; hardship in childhood, (poverty, alcoholism, etc.); and previous work experience, (nurses training). Less frequently mentioned were coming from a large family, having other children, and having a handicap. In addition to life experiences, sixteen parents stated that their religious beliefs definitely affected how they were able to cope. For example: "We were approached with the idea of taking her home, put her in a home or disconnect her. She's here because of our beliefs. Our beliefs give us strength." No parents reported their reliance on their religious beliefs as a change from before the child's condition. There were no "fox hole" conversions nor was there decreased involvement as a result. If religious beliefs were important before the child's condition, they remained so and vice versa. Participation in church activities was not as important as parents' personal faith and beliefs.

In addition to life experiences and personal beliefs, there were also specific strategies which parents used to cope on a day-to-day basis with the nurses. Inadequate or inappropriate care was always dealt with by firing the nurse immediately. The non-health related problems were dealt with by most parents (72%) becoming less tolerant of certain behaviors and becoming more assertive about confronting nurses directly. Two families totally eliminated home care nursing and eight other families replaced whole agencies and started over with new agencies. Other parents coped with problems with the nurses by not doing anything at all. They admitted to swallowing their feel-

ings and just "accept that that is the way it is." These parents felt
they needed the nurses in their home and could not risk losing them
because they "made waves." Other specific strategies families used
to help prevent or deal with problems with nurses included: regular
meetings between parents and home care staff; clearly defined orientation and training sessions for nurses including re-training of nurses
by parents when needed; a communication notebook; spending more
time talking with individual nurses to stay informed on how things
were going; and to "recognize when we enter that room (child's)—
we share responsibilities, we respect what the nurse has to say as they
do us. Everyone walks on eggs together."

An important issue mentioned by 75% of the mothers was that
they made a mistake early in home care by befriending the nurses
and trying to include them as "members of the family." These mothers
emphasized that this ultimately turned out to be negative even though
initially they felt they relied emotionally and socially on the support
of the nurses to get through the difficult early days. The problems
came later as parents became more confident and more assertive
about their authority and control over the child and the family life.
In that regard, one of the recurrent pieces of advice that experienced
parents had for parents new to home care was:

> When you are living in an abnormal situation you need to try and make
> things as normal as possible. Set rules. You can't really get close to
> the nurses and still have an employer/employee relationship. Don't
> ever forget the working relationship because that's why the nurses are
> here—to work with the child, not to socialize.

Unlike learning to cope with the nurses, parents were much less
able to identify specific strategies for how they dealt with the other
stressors and the effects of stress. In all areas the responses conveyed
the need to "accept the situation as it is because there is nothing else
to do" and a "take it one day at a time" approach. For example:

> Sometimes I don't sleep. There isn't a heck of a lot that you can do.
> There just isn't. I sit back and think about it and say to myself, 'what
> can I change? ' When there is so much, your back is against the wall.
> I simply have to take it as it comes, but it is scary. . . .

> I used to worry but I just can't any more—I juggle things—if they
> want to kick me out, fine. I get tired of being a charity case all the
> time—I hate it. You just have to go with the flow.

Parents were asked if there was anything they felt they currently
needed to help them better cope with the home care experience.

Sixteen parents (57%) cited a variety of possibilities, including: more stable and reliable home health nursing services; concrete help so parents could get out of the house (babysitters and "homemaker" services, such as help with laundry or groceries); more secure funding; counseling; and a parent support group.

No matter what the specific area, parents struggled with how to respond to questions regarding coping. With the exception of dealing with the nurses, there were no concrete strategies the parents could identify which helped them to cope with the stresses of home care. In reviewing the information on how parents perceive themselves as coping with the home care, two basic themes emerged: "take it one day at a time" and "you 'gotta' do what you 'gotta' do." Two other aspects of coping also came across: reliance on self and the immediate family for problem solving and having faith in God. Unfortunately, none of these probably can be taught to new parents entering into home care as had been the hope of the researcher. Parents stated frequently and in almost all circumstances that they dealt with different stresses in home care by "accepting what cannot be changed and changing what could." The following advice which veteran parents had for families new to home care is illustrative of how they maintain mental health through it all:

> It does get better—don't count the first month, and if you can get through the first six months you can get through anything.

> Take it one day at a time; deal with today, today and worry about tomorrow, tomorrow.

> (You) first have to be very strong-willed. (You) should know right from the beginning that there are few rewards in it, but the rewards are fantastic. It is no bed of roses because when you get tired, there isn't anybody to help you here sometimes. But it's the satisfaction of knowing that you had that child home that will get you through.

> Parents are not God—you can only bear so much. You need to look at how much you really can do. Assess the needs of the whole family— how much will it handicap providing for the needs of other kids. You can't sacrifice everyone for one.

One last, sage piece of wisdom stated by several parents:

> You can know 'better' what it might be like to be at home but you really cannot know what it will be like until you actually go home.

IMPLICATIONS AND CONCLUSIONS

In considering the process and content of this study, two salient points stand out: the great amount of data about stress must be seen in the light of the overwhelming endorsement by parents of home care of the ventilated child; and the families in this study literally learned to "do" home care on their own as there was virtually no help with problem-solving provided by anyone *after* discharge. In spite of all of the stresses and the changes the families had to endure, the families seemed to have remained committed to home care. That is both heartening and humbling. For the most part, families have made the necessary adjustments to maintain their own sanity which speaks well for the resilience and flexibility of the human spirit in the face of adversity. The challenge of this study, then, rests in finding ways to use the information obtained to enable the health care system to complement and support the existing strength of the families.

First, the immediate problems identified by the study indicate a need to provide more comprehensive planning/training/educational opportunities during the discharge process to help family members prepare for the practical aspects of living with technology in the home. The discharge planning process must include all members of the family and should address issues such as the stress of having care providers in the home, the financial present and future and the effects of the day-to-day stresses associated with technology dependence on family functioning including employment, relationships, and activities.

Secondly, the study draws attention to the cause and effect relationship of emotional aspects of home care. While the issues of denial, anger, depression, chronic sorrow, loss of freedom and so forth are not significantly different from that which other families experience, there is an intensity which is different because of the presence of care providers. Of particular concern must be the other children in the family. Siblings may be the invisible victims in home care and they, more than any of the others, felt isolated and abandoned through the home care experience.

Thirdly, vocational and independent living has not been a focus of attention in home care of the ventilated child. It seems that the intense focus on the medical condition has served to socially and emotionally handicap children and families and to discourage looking at the long term nature of the situation. Group homes, semi-independent living cooperatives and pediatric rehabilitation facilities are much needed to help the ventilated children to "leave home" in a safe manner and to have a sense of future. In turn, this "hope for independence" could help meet the developmental needs of the child and the family and help alleviate some of the helplessness which stems from the sense of role captivity inherent in such a circumstance.

Therefore, it is recommended that each family be provided the services of a community based social worker as part of the discharge plan. The purpose would include but not be limited to: 1) supporting the family in problem solving and advocacy; 2) providing a therapeutic relationship to help negotiate individual and/or family difficulties in adjusting to home care; and 3) helping the family to network within the community for the purpose of identifying, accessing and generating the resources necessary to meet the needs of the family, e.g., educational programming, volunteers to help with the other children, service groups to help provide materials and labor for environmental modifications and/or opportunities for special activities, etc. Social work, advocacy, or other mental health services in the community are not now reimbursed by private or public funding agencies as a justifiable cost of home care. Such a change would require state as well as federal commitment to mental health as it relates to physical health.

On an even larger scale, there are important policies which affect home care once the technology dependent child reaches age 21. Although care of disabled adults at home affects far greater numbers of individuals than pediatric home care, few of the services available to children are available to adults. When these children turn 21, the paucity of adult services is potentially devastating because services which exist for children will be removed when the magic age of 21 is reached. It makes no logical sense in the context of society that those with the most family resources (children) receive so many services while the disabled adult and elderly populations with far fewer family and social supports receive almost no services. The disparity between adult and child resources requires a national health and home care policy which looks at the life span of the disabled individual. Children become adults and the reality of potential stress of the adult life for the ventilated individual makes the stress of dealing with nurses minor and trivial by comparison. There is the need for changes with regard to Medicaid and Medicare reimbursement for care in the home with a more logical and equitable distribution of resources across the life span.

REFERENCES

Barbarin, O. A., Hughes, D., & Chesler, M. A. (1985). Stress, coping, and marital functioning among parents of children with cancer. *Journal of Marriage and the Family, 47*, 473–80.

Blacher, J. (1984). A dynamic perspective on the impact of a severely handicapped child on the family. In J. Blacher (Ed.), *Severely handicapped young children and their families* (pp. 3–50). London: Academic Press, Inc.

Brown, B. (1984). *Between health and illness*. MA: Houghton and Mifflin.

Coffman, S. P. (1983). Parents' perceptions of needs for themselves and their children in a cerebral palsy clinic. *Issues in Comprehensive Pediatric Nursing, 6*, 67–77.

Featherstone, H. (1980). *A difference in the family: Living with a disabled child*. NY: Basic Books.

Feinberg, E. A. (1986). Family stress in pediatric home care. *Caring, 4(5)*, 39–41.

Frederick, W. N. & Frederick, W. L. (1981). Psychosocial assets of parents of handicapped and nonhandicapped children. *American Journal of Mental Deficiency, 85*, 551–553.

Goldberg, A., Faure, E., & Vaughn, C. (1984). Home care for life supported persons: An approach to program development. *Journal of Pediatrics, 104*, 785–795.

Hamburg, B. A. (1974). Early adolescence: a specific and stressful stage of the life cycle. In G. Coelho, D. Hamburg, & J. Adams (Eds.), *Coping and adaptation* (pp. 101–124). NY: Basic Books, Inc.

Hodges, L. C. & Parker, J. (1987). Concerns of parents with diabetic children. *Pediatric Nursing, 13*, 22–24, 68.

Horner, M. M., Rawlins, P. & Giles, K. (1987). How parents of children with chronic conditions perceive their own needs. *Maternal and Child Nursing, 12*, 40–43.

Litt, I. F., Cuskey, W. R., & Rosenberg, A. (1982). Role of self-esteem and autonomy in determining medication compliance among adolescents with juvenile rheumatoid arthritis. *Pediatrics, 69*, 15–17.

Lyon, S., & Preis, A. (1983). Working with families of severely handicapped person. In M. Seligman (Ed.), *The family with a handicapped child* (pp. 203–234). NY: Grune and Stratton.

McCubbin, H. I. & Patterson, J. M. (1983). Family transitions: adaptation to stress. In H. I. McCubbin & C. R. Figley (Eds.), *Stress and the family: Coping with normative transitions (Vol. 1)*. NY: Brunner/Mazel.

McCubbin, M. (1984). Nursing assessment of parental coping with cystic fibrosis. *Western Journal of Nursing Research, 6*, 407–418.

McHale, S. M., Simeonsson, R. J. & Sloan, J. L. (1984). Children with handicapped brothers and sisters. In E. Schopler & G. Mesibov (Eds.), *The effects of autism on the family* (pp. 327–342). NY: Plenum.

McKeever, P. (1983). Siblings of chronically ill children: a literature review with implications for research and practice. *American Journal of Orthopsychiatry, 53*, 209–218.

Office of Technology Assessment (OTA). (1987). *Technology dependent children: Hospital vs home care*. Technical Memorandum. US Congress, Washington, D.C. #OTA-TM-H-38.

Powell, T. & Ogle, P. (1985). *Brothers and sisters—A special part of exceptional families*. Baltimore: Paul H. Brookes Publishing Co.

Reynolds, J. M., Gerralda, M. E., Jameson, R. A., & Postlethwaite, R. J. (1986). Living with chronic renal failure. *Child: Care, Health, and Development, 12*, 401–407.

Shonkoff, J. P., Jarman, F. C., & Kohlenberg, T. M. (1987). Family transitions, crises, and adaptations. *Current Problems in Pediatrics*. Illinois: Year Book Medical Publishers, Inc., *17*, 501–553.

Stuifbergen, A. K. (1987). The impact of chronic illness on families. *Family and Community Health, 9*, 43–51.

Travis, G. (1976). *Chronic illness in children: Its impact on child and family*. CA: Stanford University Press.

Treiber, F., Mabe III, P. A., & Wilson, G. (1987). Psychological adjustment of sickle cell children and their siblings. *Journal of Children's Health Care, 16*, 82–88.

Turner, R. J. (1983). Direct, indirect, and moderating effects of social support on psychological distress and associated conditions. In H. B. Kaplan (Ed.), *Psychological stress: Trends in theory and research* (pp. 105–155). NY: Academic Press.

Weinstock, N. (1986). The family of the high risk infant. In E. Ahmann (Ed.), *Home care for the high risk infant: A holistic guide to using technology* (pp. 293–306). MD: Aspen Publications.

Yoos, L. (1987). Chronic childhood illnesses: developmental issues. *Pediatric Nursing, 13*, 25–28.

Section IX
Resources

CHAPTER 19

A NATIONWIDE DIRECTORY OF RESOURCES FOR MEDICALLY COMPLEX CHILDREN

ANN HOLMAN
NEIL J. HOCHSTADT
DIANE M. YOST

INTRODUCTION

Medically complex children, their families, caretakers, and the professionals who work with them, often have need for additional information and support. To the best of our knowledge there is no single compendium of resources for medically complex children. This chapter attempts to provide such a resource for those who care for, and work with, medically complex children. The directory reflects the diverse health care needs of this population of children as well as the wide range of services, disciplines, facilities and organizations involved in their care. The resources included are for informational value; inclusion does not imply our endorsement. We have attempted to make this directory as complete as possible. However, given the rapid increase in this population, its diversity, and the ever growing resources available, this directory may not be as complete as we would like. We invite readers to contact us with additional resources. We hope to update this directory periodically.

HOSPITAL PROGRAMS FOR MEDICALLY COMPLEX AND VENTILATOR DEPENDENT CHILDREN

Cardinal Glennon Hospital
1465 S. Grand
St. Louis, MO 63104

Children's Hospital of Los Angeles
4650 Sunset Blvd.
Los Angeles, CA 90027

Children's Hospital of New Orleans
200 Henry Clay
New Orleans, LA 70118

Children's Hospital of Orange County
P.O. Box 5700
Orange, CA 92668

Children's Hospital of Philadelphia
34th & Civic Center Blvd.
Philadelphia, PA 19104

Children's Memorial Hospital
2300 Children's Plaza
Chicago, IL 60614

Hospital for Sick Children
1731 Bunker Hill Road, N.E.
Washington, D.C. 20017

La Rabida Children's Hospital and Research Center
East 65th Street at Lake Michigan
Chicago, IL 60649

Mott Children's Hospital
University of Michigan Medical Center
Ann Arbor, MI 48109

Pediatric Pulmonary Care
University of Washington
Department of Pediatrics
Seattle, WA 98195

Riley Hospital for Children
702 Barnhill Drive
Indianapolis, IN 46223

St. Louis Children's Hospital
400 S. Kings Highway
St. Louis, MO 63110

University Hospital
University of Wisconsin
600 Highland Avenue
Madison, WI 53712

INTERMEDIATE, LONG-TERM AND RESIDENTIAL PROGRAMS FOR MEDICALLY COMPLEX AND VENTILATOR DEPENDENT CHILDREN

Broward Children's Center
200 SE 19th Avenue
Pompano Beach, FL 33060

Cumberland Hospital
P.O. Box 150
New Kent, VA 23124

New Medico Head Injury System
(Home Office)
(also accepts ventilator dependent children)
113 Broad Street
Lynn, MA 01902
New Medico has facilities throughout the country

Vencor, Inc. (Home Office)
Brown and Williamson Tower
Suite 700
Louisville, KY 40202

Vencor has 9 facilities throughout the country:
Mansville, TX
Dallas, TX
San Antonio, TX
Fort Lauderdale, FL
Tampa, FL
Gonzales, LA
Youngstown, AR
Sycamore, IL
La Grange, IN

RESPITE INFORMATION

Texas Respite Resource Network
P.O. Box 7330
San Antonio, TX 78207

CASE MANAGEMENT

**Coordinating Center for Home
and Community Care**
P.O. Box 613
Severn Professional Building
Millersville, MD 21108

**Division of Services for Crippled
Children**
University of Illinois
1919 W. Taylor Street
Chicago, IL 60612

**R.E.A.C.H. (Rural Efforts to
Assist Children at Home)**
Institute for Child Health Policy
5100 S.W. 34th Street, Suite 323
Gainesville, FL 32608

**SKIP (Sick Kids Need Involved
People)**
500 E. 83rd Street, Apt. 1B
New York, N.Y. 10028

**Ventilator Assisted Care Program
of Louisiana Children's Hospital**
200 Henry Clay Avenue
New Orleans, Louisiana 70118

NATIONAL ORGANIZATIONS FOR INFORMATION AND ADVOCACY

American Bar Association
Child Advocacy Center
1800 M St. N.W., Suite 200
Washington, D.C. 20036

**Association for the Care of
Children's Health**
7910 Woodmont Avenue,
Suite 300
Bethesda, MD 20814

**Canadian Rehabilitation Council
for the Disabled**
One Yonge Street, Suite 2110
Toronto, Ontario, Canada M5E 1E5

Challenge International
6719 Lowell Avenue
McLean, VA 22101

Children's Defense Fund
122 C Street, N.W., Suite 400
Washington, D.C. 20001

**Coalition on Sexuality and
Disability, Inc.**
380 2nd Avenue
4th Floor
New York, N.Y. 10010

**Congress of Organizations of the
Physically Handicapped**
1660 Beverly Avenue
Tinley Park, IL 60477-1904

**Disability Rights Education and
Defense Fund, Inc.**
1616 P St., N.W.
Suite 100
Washington, D.C. 20036

**Disability Rights Education and
Defense Fund, Inc.**
2212 Sixth Street
Berkeley, CA 94710

**International Shriners
Headquarters**
2900 Rocky Point
Tampa, FL 33607

National Center for Education in Maternal and Child Care
38th & R Streets, N.W.
Georgetown University
Washington, D.C. 20057

National Center for Youth with Disabilities
Adolescent Health Program
University of Minnesota
Box 721—UMHC
Harvard Street/East River Road
Minneapolis, MN 54455

National Maternal and Child Health Resource Center
Julie Beckett, Dept. P.
University of Iowa
College of Law
Iowa City, Iowa, 52242

National Easter Seal Society
2023 W. Ogden Ave.
Chicago, IL 60612

National Organization on Disability
910 16th Street, NW
Washington, D.C. 20006

National Self-Help Clearinghouse
33 W. 42nd Street
New York, N.Y. 10036

SKIP (Sick Kids Need Involved People)
500 E. 83rd Street, Apt. 1B
New York, N.Y. 10028

GOVERNMENT AGENCIES

Administration on Developmental Disabilities
Department of Health and Human Services
200 Independence Ave., S.W.
336E Humphrey Blvd.
Washington, D.C. 20201

Closer Look/Parents' Campaign for Handicapped Children
1201 16th Street, Suite 233
Washington, D.C. 20036

Department of Health and Human Services
Division of Children, Youth and Families
330 C Street, S.W.
Washington, D.C. 20201

Maternal and Child Health Bureau
Health Resources and Services Administration
Public Health Service
5600 Fishers Lane, Room 9-11
Rockville, MD 20857

National Information Center for Children & Youth with Handicaps
P.O. Box 1492
Washington, D.C. 20013

National Institutes of Health
National Institute of Child Health and Human Development
Bldg. 31, Room 2A03
9000 Rockville Pike
Bethesda, MD 20892

National Health Information Center
Office of Disease Prevention and Health Protection (ODPHP)
P.O. Box 1133
Washington, D.C. 20013-1133

Office of Special Education and Rehabilitation Services
Clearinghouse on the Handicapped
U.S. Department of Education
330 E. Street, S.W.
Switzer Building
Washington, D.C. 20202

President's Committee on Employment of the Handicapped
1111 20 Street, N.W.
Room 636
Washington, D.C. 20036

CHILD WELFARE ORGANIZATIONS

American Public Welfare Association
1125 Fifteenth Street, N.W.
Suite 300
Washington, D.C. 20005

Child Welfare League of America
440 First Street, N.W.
Washington, D.C. 20001

Child Welfare Training Institute
Center of Social Policy and
    Community Development
Temple University
1500 N. Broadway Street
Philadelphia, PA 19122

National Adoption Center
1218 Chestnut Street
Philadelphia, PA 19107

National Institute for Alternative Care Professionals
10100 Elida Road
Delphos, OH 45833

National Resource Center of Child Welfare Service
Suite S. 200
1800 M. Street, N.W.
Washington, D.C. 20036

National Resource Center on Family Based Services
240 Oakdale Hall
Iowa City, IA

National Resource Center for Foster and Institutional Care
Child Welfare Institute
Station C
P.O. Box 77364
Atlanta, GA 30357

National Resource Center for Special Needs Adoption
P.O. 337
Chelsea, MI 48118

North American Council on Adoptable Children
P.O. Box 14808
Minneapolis, MN 55414

EDUCATION

Task Force on Children with Special Health Conditions
Association for the Care of
    Children's Health *and*
The National Center for Training
    Caregivers
Children's Hospital
200 Henry Clay Avenue
New Orleans, Louisiana 70118

Division of Physically Handicapped
Council for Exceptional Children
1920 Association Drive
Reston, VA 22091-1589

INNOVATIVE PROGRAMS FOR MEDICALLY COMPLEX CHILDREN

Broward Children's Center
200 S.E. 19th Ave.
Pompano Beach, FL 30060
(Mailing Address:
    P.O. Box 3248
    Pompano Beach, FL 33072)

Children's Crisis Center, Inc.
655 West 8th Street
Jacksonville, FL 32209

Leake and Watts Children's Home
463 Hawthorne Avenue
Yonkers, N.Y. 10705

**Prescribed Pediatric Extended
  Care, Inc.**
4131 N.W. 28th Lane, Suite 3A
Gainesville, FL 32606

Project Impact
25 West Street
Boston, MA 02111

OTHER RESOURCES

Exceptional Parent magazine's yearly September issue—a complete listing
of organizations devoted to assisting those with special medical conditions
(P.O. Box 3000, Denville, N.J. 07834)

INDEX

Note: Page numbers followed by f indicate figures; page numbers followed by t indicate tables.